Advanced Heart Failure

Editors

JAMES C. FANG
MICHAEL M. GIVERTZ

HEART FAILURE CLINICS

www.heartfailure.theclinics.com

Consulting Editors
MANDEEP R. MEHRA
JAVED BUTLER

Founding Editor
JAGAT NARULA

July 2016 • Volume 12 • Number 3

ELSEVIER

1600 John F. Kennedy Boulevard • Suite 1800 • Philadelphia, Pennsylvania, 19103-2899

http://www.theclinics.com

HEART FAILURE CLINICS Volume 12, Number 3
July 2016 ISSN 1551-7136, ISBN-13: 978-0-323-44846-8

Editor: Lauren Boyle
Developmental Editor: Alison Swety

Heart Failure Clinics (ISSN 1551-7136) is published quarterly by Elsevier Inc., 360 Park Avenue South, New York, NY 10010-1710. Months of publication are January, April, July, and October. Business and editorial offices: 1600 John F. Kennedy Boulevard, Suite 1800, Philadelphia, PA 19103-2899. Periodicals postage paid at New York, NY, and additional mailing offices. Subscription prices are USD 240.00 per year for US individuals, USD 431.00 per year for US institutions, USD 100.00 per year for US students and residents, USD 280.00 per year for Canadian individuals, USD 499.00 per year for Canadian institutions, USD 300.00 per year for international individuals, USD 499.00 per year for international institutions, and USD 100.00 per year for Canadian and foreign students/residents. To receive student and resident rate, orders must be accompanied by name of affiliated institution, date of term, and the *signature* of program/residency coordinator on institution letterhead. Orders will be billed at individual rate until proof of status is received. Foreign air speed delivery is included in all *Clinics* subscription prices. All prices are subject to change without notice. **POSTMASTER:** Send address changes to *Heart Failure Clinics*, Elsevier Health Sciences Division, Subscription Customer Service, 3251 Riverport Lane, Maryland Heights, MO 63043. **Customer Service: 1-800-654-2452 (US and Canada). From outside of the US and Canada, call 314-447-8871. Fax: 314-447-8029. For print support, E-mail: JournalsCustomerService-usa@elsevier.com. For online support, E-mail: JournalsOnlineSupport-usa@elsevier.com.**

Reprints. For copies of 100 or more of articles in this publication, please contact the Commercial Reprints Department, Elsevier Inc., 360 Park Avenue South, New York, NY 10010-1710. Tel.: 212-633-3874; Fax: 212-633-3820; E-mail: reprints@elsevier.com.

Heart Failure Clinics is covered in *MEDLINE/PubMed (Index Medicus)*.

Contributors

CONSULTING EDITORS

MANDEEP R. MEHRA, MD, FACC, FACP, FRCP
Heart and Vascular Center, Brigham and Women's Hospital, Harvard Medical School, Boston, Massachusetts

JAVED BUTLER, MD, MPH, MBA
Stony Brook University Heart Institute, Department of Internal Medicine, Stony Brook School of Medicine, Stony Brook University Medical Center, Stony Brook, New York

EDITORS

JAMES C. FANG, MD
Professor of Medicine and Executive Director, Cardiovascular Service Line, Division of Cardiovascular Medicine, University of Utah Health Science Center, Salt Lake City, Utah

MICHAEL M. GIVERTZ, MD
Cardiovascular Division, Department of Medicine, Brigham and Women's Hospital, Harvard Medical School, Boston, Massachusetts

AUTHORS

JESSICA L. BROWN, MD
Houston Methodist Hospital, Houston, Texas

VALENTINA CARUBELLI, MD
Cardiology, Department of Medical and Surgical Specialties, Radiological Sciences and Public Health, University of Brescia, Brescia, Italy

SUNIT-PREET CHAUDHRY, MD
Department of Medicine, Center for Advanced Heart Disease, Brigham and Women's Hospital, Harvard Medical School, Boston, Massachusetts

ANTHONY J. CHOI, MD
Electrophysiology Laboratory, Cardiac Arrhythmia Service, Cardiology Division, Department of Medicine, Massachusetts General Hospital, Harvard Medical School, Boston, Massachusetts

JENNIFER A. COWGER, MD, MS
Director of MCS Research, St. Vincent Heart Center of Indiana, Indianapolis, Indiana

STAVROS G. DRAKOS, MD, PhD
Molecular Medicine Program, Eccles Institute of Human Genetics and UTAH Cardiac

Transplant Program, Division of Cardiovascular Medicine, University of Utah School of Medicine, Salt Lake City, Utah

JERRY D. ESTEP, MD
Associate Professor of Clinical Cardiology, Medical Director, Heart Transplant and LVAD Program, Section Head of Heart Transplant and Mechanical Circulatory Support, Division of Heart Failure, Houston Methodist Institute of Academic Medicine, Methodist DeBakey Heart and Vascular Center, Houston Methodist Hospital, Houston, Texas

AMANDA J. FAVREAU-LESSARD, PhD
Research Fellow, Center for Molecular Medicine, Maine Medical Center Research Institute, Maine Medical Center, Scarborough, Maine

PETER C. FERRIN, BA
Molecular Medicine Program, University of Utah, Salt Lake City, Utah

JILL M. GELOW, MD, MPH
Assistant Professor of Medicine, Heart Failure, Heart Transplant and Advanced Cardiac Devices; Knight Cardiovascular Institute, Oregon Health and Science University, Portland, Oregon

Contributors

MAHAZARIN GINWALLA, MD, MS
Department of Cardiovascular Medicine,
Harrington Heart and Vascular Institute,
University Hospitals Case Medical Center,
Cleveland, Ohio

ELIO GORGA, MD
Cardiology, Department of Medical and
Surgical Specialties, Radiological Sciences
and Public Health, University of Brescia,
Brescia, Italy

EMER JOYCE, MD, PhD
Staff Physician, Section of Heart Failure and
Cardiac Transplant Medicine, Robert and
Suzanne Tomsich, Department of
Cardiovascular Medicine, Sydell and Arnold
Miller Family Heart and Vascular Institute,
Cleveland Clinic Foundation, Cleveland, Ohio

MICHELLE M. KITTLESON, MD, PhD
Associate Professor of Medicine,
Cedars-Sinai, Division of Cardiology,
Cedars-Sinai Heart Institute, Los Angeles,
California

CARLO LOMBARDI, MD
Cardiology, Department of Medical and
Surgical Specialties, Radiological Sciences
and Public Health, University of Brescia,
Brescia, Italy

LAUREN McCREATH, BA
Molecular Medicine Program, University of
Utah, Salt Lake City, Utah

ROBERT J. MENTZ, MD
Duke University Medical Center, Duke Clinical
Research Institute, Durham, North Carolina

MARCO METRA, MD
Cardiology, Department of Medical and
Surgical Specialties, Radiological Sciences
and Public Health, University of Brescia,
Brescia, Italy

JAMES O. MUDD, MD
Associate Professor of Medicine, Heart Failure,
Heart Transplant and Advanced Cardiac
Devices; Knight Cardiovascular Institute,
Oregon Health and Science University,
Portland, Oregon

SUTIP NAVANKASATTUSAS, PhD
Division of Cardiovascular Medicine, University
of Utah School of Medicine, Molecular
Medicine Program, Eccles Institute of Human
Genetics and UTAH Cardiac Transplant
Program, Salt Lake City, Utah

AKSHAY PENDYAL, MD
Fellow, Cardiovascular Medicine; Knight
Cardiovascular Institute, Oregon Health and
Science University, Portland, Oregon

CARRIE PUCKETT, DO
Fellow, Advanced Heart Failure and Transplant
Cardiology; Knight Cardiovascular Institute,
Oregon Health and Science University,
Portland, Oregon

ALICE RAVERA, MD
Cardiology, Department of Medical and
Surgical Specialties, Radiological Sciences
and Public Health, University of Brescia,
Brescia, Italy

SERGEY RYZHOV, MD, PhD
Faculty Scientist, Center for Molecular
Medicine, Maine Medical Center Research
Institute, Scarborough, Maine

DOUGLAS B. SAWYER, MD, PhD
Chief of Cardiovascular Services, Maine
Medical Center, Portland, Maine; Faculty
Scientist, Center for Molecular Medicine,
Maine Medical Center Research Institute,
Maine Medical Center, Scarborough, Maine

JAGMEET P. SINGH, MD, DPhil
Electrophysiology Laboratory, Cardiac
Arrhythmia Service, Cardiology Division,
Department of Medicine, Massachusetts
General Hospital, Harvard Medical School,
Boston, Massachusetts

GARRICK C. STEWART, MD
Department of Medicine, Center for Advanced
Heart Disease, Brigham and Women's
Hospital, Harvard Medical School, Boston,
Massachusetts

SUNU S. THOMAS, MD, MSc
Heart Failure and Transplant Services,
Cardiology Division, Department of
Medicine, Massachusetts General Hospital,
Harvard Medical School, Boston,
Massachusetts

MUHAMMED WAQAS, MD
St. Vincent Heart Center of Indiana,
Indianapolis, Indiana

Contents

> Heart failure is a complex clinical syndrome. The natural history of this syndrome is progressive. Advanced heart failure is present when a patient has signs and symptoms of heart failure that are refractory to therapy. Patients with the most advanced disease and worst prognosis can be identified using iterative, integrated clinical assessment of symptom burden, effort intolerance, and cardiac dysfunction. Recognizing the transition to advanced heart failure is necessary for referral to an advanced heart disease program. Advanced heart disease specialists can tailor medical therapies, perform risk stratification, and evaluate candidacy for mechanical support, transplantation, or end-of-life palliative treatment options.

> Recently, there has been increased appreciation of the identification and management of comorbidities in heart failure patients, and for therapies targeting conventional heart failure signs and symptoms. Renal dysfunction is common in patients with heart failure and is associated with high morbidity and mortality. Early identification of renal damage through novel biomarkers and the use of new pharmacological strategies aimed at preserving renal function may represent an important objective in the treatment. This article reviews the epidemiology and pathophysiology of cardiorenal syndrome in heart failure, and highlights novel biomarkers and improved therapies targeting renal dysfunction.

> Liver disease is a common sequela of heart failure and can range from mild reversible liver injury to hepatic fibrosis and, in its most severe form, cardiac cirrhosis. Hepatic fibrosis and cirrhosis due to chronic heart failure have important implications for prognosis, medication management, mechanical circulatory support, and heart transplantation. This article reviews the current understanding of liver disease in heart failure and provides a framework for approaching liver disease in the advanced heart failure population.

> Frailty is defined as a biological syndrome reflecting impaired physiologic reserve and heightened vulnerability to stressors. The evolving profile of heart failure (HF), increased survival of aging patients with complex comorbidities in parallel with the growing population undergoing mechanical circulatory support as lifetime therapy,

means that advanced HF specialists are becoming aware of the burden of frailty and its downstream consequences on postintervention outcomes in these patients. The limited data available to date suggest that frailty is highly prevalent in patients with advanced HF and appears to provide prognostic information not captured by traditional risk assessment.

primary graft dysfunction, and advances in the management of sensitized heart transplant candidates. Developments in these areas may result in more equitable distribution and expansion of the donor pool and improved quality of life and survival for heart transplant recipients.

Patients with advanced heart failure are at high risk for progression of their disease and sudden cardiac death. The role of device therapy in this patient population continues to evolve and is directed toward improving cardiac pump function and/or reducing sudden arrhythmic death.

Heart failure is a leading case of morbidity and mortality worldwide, and patients with advanced heart failure have limited options without any available cure. These options mainly include cardiac transplantation or mechanical circulatory support device implantation. Chronic home inotropes are an option in these patients for a variety of indications. This report discusses the use of chronic home inotropes in palliated heart failure patients and reviews the role of palliative care management in end-stage heart failure.

Adverse myocardial remodeling can be reversed by medical, surgical, and device therapies leading to reduced heart failure (HF) morbidity and mortality and significant improvements in the structure and function of the failing heart. The growing population of HF patients who experience a degree of myocardial improvement should be better studied in terms of long-term outcomes and underlying biology to more clearly define the difference between recovery and remission. These investigations should also be focused in determining whether in chronic HF patients complete myocardial recovery is achievable at a meaningful rate and help us better understand, predict, and manipulate cardiac recovery.

Recovery of ventricular function occurs in a subset of patients with advanced heart failure treated with medical and/or mechanical therapy. Finding strategies that induce ventricular recovery through induction of repair, regeneration, or "rejuvenation" is a long-sought goal of research programs. Cell-based strategies, use of recombinant growth and survival factors, and gene delivery are under investigation. In this brief article we highlight a few of the biological approaches in development to treat heart failure.

HEART FAILURE CLINICS

THE CLINICS ARE AVAILABLE ONLINE!
Access your subscription at:
www.theclinics.com

Preface

Advanced Therapies for Advanced Heart Failure: Time to Raise Awareness

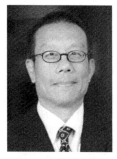
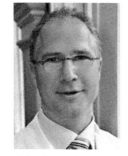

James C. Fang, MD   Michael M. Givertz, MD

Editors

The past quarter century has seen tremendous progress in the treatment of heart failure (**Box 1**). As recently as 1990, the majority of ambulatory patients were managed with digoxin, diuretics, and vasodilators, while heart transplant was available only for a select few. With the understanding of the importance of neurohumoral activation on disease progression came the introduction of renin-angiotensin-aldosterone system inhibitors and β-blockers, which had a marked impact on survival. Device-based therapies to prevent sudden death and resynchronize the heart added further to therapeutic progress. More recently, evolution in mechanical circulatory support has brought both temporary and longer-term solutions for patients with end-stage heart disease.[1]

Despite these advances, it is estimated that nearly 6 million Americans are living with chronic heart failure, and up to 250,000 suffer from advanced disease, defined as the presence of progressive and/or persistent severe signs and symptoms of heart failure despite optimized medical, surgical, and device therapy.[2] It is important to identify patients with advanced heart failure because morbidity is progressive and survival is often short. Quality of life and daily activities are further limited by older age, frailty, and comorbidities. Psychosocial and economic constraints may also affect a patient's ability to access and benefit from optimal care. For these high-risk patients and their providers, an updated understanding of pathophysiology and novel treatment strategies are needed.

> **Box 1**
> **Therapies available for the treatment of chronic heart failure in 1990 and 2015**
>
> *Twenty-five years of progress in heart failure*
>
> | 1990 | 2015 |
> |------|------|
> | • Digoxin | • ACEI/ARB/β-blockers |
> | • Diuretics | • Aldosterone antagonists |
> | • Vasodilators | • ARNI, ivabradine |
> | • Transplant | • ICD/CRT |
> | | • PAP monitor (CardioMEMs) |
> | | • LVAD/BIVAD/PVAD |
> | | • Disease management |
> | | • Palliative care |
>
> *Abbreviations:* ACEI, angiotensin-converting enzyme inhibitor; ARB, angiotensin receptor blocker; ARNI, angiotensin receptor neprilysin inhibitor; BIVAD, biventricular assist device; CRT, cardiac resynchronization therapy; ICD, implantable cardioverter-defibrillator; LVAD, left ventricular assist device; PAP, pulmonary artery pressure; PVAD, percutaneous ventricular assist device.

For this special issue of *Heart Failure Clinics*, we invited leaders in the heart failure community to provide critical updates in the contemporary understanding of advanced heart failure. Important topics include epidemiology, pathophysiology, medical and device-based therapies, and end-of-life care. Clinical insights into myocardial recovery

Heart Failure Clin 12 (2016) ix–x
http://dx.doi.org/10.1016/j.hfc.2016.05.001
1551-7136/16/$ – see front matter © 2016 Published by Elsevier Inc.

and novel biological therapies are also provided. While consensus guidelines to manage heart failure exist,[3] these documents are infrequently published, slow to be updated, and typically do not have the "authority" to go beyond randomized clinical trials. Level of evidence C (or expert opinion) is needed to fill in the knowledge gaps and provide clinicians with individual pathways for care. Our hope is that the current compendium of expert opinion succeeds in these goals.

James C. Fang, MD
Division of Cardiovascular Medicine
University of Utah Health Science Center
30 North 1900 East, Room 4A100
Salt Lake City, UT 84132, USA

Michael M. Givertz, MD
Cardiovascular Division
Brigham and Women's Hospital
75 Francis Street
Boston, MA 02115, USA

E-mail addresses:
james.fang@hsc.utah.edu (J.C. Fang)
mgivertz@partners.org (M.M. Givertz)

REFERENCES

1. Stewart GC, Givertz MM. Mechanical circulatory support for advanced heart failure: patients and technology in evolution. Circulation 2012;125: 1304–15.
2. Fang JC, Ewald GA, Allen LA, et al. Advanced (stage D) heart failure: a statement from the Heart Failure Society of America guidelines committee. J Card Fail 2015;21:519–34.
3. Yancy CW, Jessup M, Bozkurt B, et al. 2013 ACCF/AHA guideline for the management of heart failure: a report of the American College of Cardiology Foundation/American Heart Association Task Force on practice guidelines. Circulation 2013;128: e240–319.

Advanced Heart Failure
Prevalence, Natural History, and Prognosis

Sunit-Preet Chaudhry, MD, Garrick C. Stewart, MD*

KEYWORDS

- Heart failure • Cardiomyopathy • Prognosis • Risk assessment • Clinical decision making

KEY POINTS

- Advanced heart failure is defined by the presence of progressive and/or persistent severe symptoms despite optimized medical, surgical, and device therapy.
- Overlapping classification schemes—New York Heart Association class, ACC (American College of Cardiology)/American Heart Association stages, and Interagency Registry for Mechanically Assisted Circulatory Support profiles—provide complementary descriptive information for patients with advanced heart disease.
- In select patients, early recognition of advanced heart failure facilitates the timely deployment of surgical heart failure therapies in the context of patient-centered shared decision making.
- Risk stratification in advanced heart failure can be informed by clinical history, physical examination, routine blood tests, assessment of functional capacity, and cardiac imaging.

INTRODUCTION

Heart failure is a complex clinical syndrome resulting from impairment of ventricular filling or ejection of blood associated with symptoms of dyspnea, fatigue, and peripheral and/or pulmonary edema.[1] Although there have been dramatic innovations in medical and device treatments for heart failure in recent decades, the incidence of heart failure is increasing. The heart failure syndrome affects an estimated 5.7 million Americans and more than 23 million people worldwide.[2,3] The heart failure epidemic has a staggering impact on quality of life, functioning, and longevity, while imposing heavy costs on the health care system. The identification of the syndrome of advanced heart failure requires an iterative clinical assessment integrating routinely available clinical risk markers. Recognizing that a patient suffers from advanced

heart failure promotes timely triage to surgical cardiac therapies, such as mechanical support or transplant, and allows clinicians to initiate the development of end-of-life care plans consistent with patient values, preferences, and goals.

The syndrome of heart failure is commonly divided into 2 categories: heart failure with reduced ejection fraction (HFrEF) and heart failure with preserved ejection fraction (HFpEF). Although past literature and guidelines have proposed varying definitions of HFrEF,[1,4,5] the American College of Cardiology Foundation/American Heart Association (ACCF/AHA) Task Force currently defines it as heart failure with an ejection fraction (EF) of no more than 40%. Patients with an EF of at least 50% make up the group of patients definitively characterized with HFpEF, while the group of patients with EF between 41% and

Disclosure: The authors report no conflicts of interest or disclosures relevant to this article.
Department of Medicine, Center for Advanced Heart Disease, Brigham and Women's Hospital, Harvard Medical School, 75 Francis Street, Boston, MA 02115, USA
* Corresponding author. Cardiovascular Division, Brigham and Women's Hospital, 75 Francis Street, Boston, MA 02115.
E-mail address: gcstewart@partners.org

Heart Failure Clin 12 (2016) 323–333
http://dx.doi.org/10.1016/j.hfc.2016.03.001
1551-7136/16/$ – see front matter © 2016 Elsevier Inc. All rights reserved.

heartfailure.theclinics.com

49% has been variably classified in clinical trials as either HFpEF or HFrEF. Although advanced disease exists in patients with HFpEF, its prevalence and prognosis remain poorly understood. Current understanding of the epidemiology and natural history of advanced heart failure has been largely derived from the systolic heart failure literature.

Multiple classification systems have been devised to characterize the severity of heart failure beyond EF alone. The earliest and most commonly used classification system is from the New York Heart Association (NYHA), which divides patients into 1 of 4 classes based on their exercise capacity and symptom burden. Within this system, patients with persistent NYHA class 4 symptoms are deemed to have advanced heart failure.[6] In 2001, the ACCF/AHA released a new system that placed emphasis on antecedent risk factors and progressive stages of disease similar to the approach commonly used in cancer staging. In this system, stage D patients were considered as advanced heart failure and were defined as having refractory heart failure despite optimal medical therapy (**Fig. 1**).

Most recently, in 2009 the Interagency Registry for Mechanically Assisted Circulatory Support (INTERMACS) classification system was developed to stratify the advanced heart failure patients undergoing consideration of mechanical circulatory support[7] (**Table 1**). The INTERMACS patient profiles are important for framing discussion surrounding the appropriateness and timing of mechanical support. In the end, the classification systems are complementary to one another, describing current symptoms (NYHA), stepwise disease progression (ACCF/AHA stages), and integrated assessment of advanced disease trajectory (INTERMACS profile). As might be expected given these evolving classification schemes and heterogenous population at risk, the major

cardiovascular societies have varying definitions of advanced heart failure (**Table 2**).[8]

PREVALENCE

Over the last 3 decades, there has been a change in the definition and prevalence of advanced heart failure as treatment options have evolved. Prior to the routine use of neurohormonal antagonists, medical therapy for advanced systolic heart failure consisted of digoxin and diuretics, with advanced heart failure defined as patients with persistent NYHA class 4 symptoms.[9] With the advent of renin-angiotensin-aldosterone antagonists and beta-blockers, as well as widespread use of implantable cardioverter–defibrillators for the primary prevention of sudden death, advanced heart failure patients today are often older at presentation and have accumulated more comorbid medical conditions. Most recently, the Heart Failure Society of America (HFSA) has defined advanced heart failure as the presence of progressive and/or persistent severe symptoms of heart failure despite optimized medical, surgical, and device therapy.[10]

Given the shifting definitions of advanced heart failure and the fact that many signs of advanced disease may be nonspecific, the true prevalence is elusive. A population-based, cross-sectional, random sample of the Olmstead County database estimated the prevalence of stage D heart failure to be only 0.2%.[11] Experts have estimated the prevalence to range widely from 6% to 25% among patients with established heart failure, with estimates influenced by the definition used and population studied.[8] Findings from the Acute Decompensated Heart Failure national registry (ADHERE) suggest that 5% of all heart failure patients have end-stage disease with refractory symptoms despite optimal medical therapy.[12] At the current time, advanced heart failure in the

AHA/ACC Stages

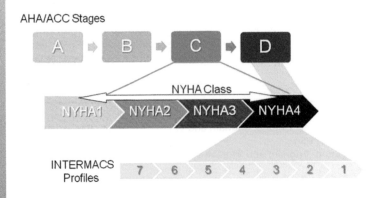

Fig. 1. Classification schemes for heart failure severity. Overlapping classification systems provide complementary descriptive and prognostic information for patients with advanced heart disease. NYHA classifies dynamic functional limitation, the American Heart Association/American College of Cardiology-Stages of Heart Failure highlight antecedent risk factors and disease progression, while the INTERMACS patient profiles integrate symptom burden and ongoing measures use to treat evolving shock.

Table 1
Interagency Registry for Mechanically Assisted Circulatory Support patient profiles

Patient Profile	Official Shorthand
1	"Crash and burn"
2	"Sliding fast" on inotropes
3	"Stable" on continuous inotropes
4	Resting symptoms on oral therapy at home
5	"Housebound", comfortable at rest but symptoms with minimum activities of daily living
6	"Walking wounded", activities of daily living possible by meaningful activity limited
7	Advanced NYHA class III

Adapted from Stevenson LW, Pagani FD, Young JB, et al. INTERMACS profiles of advanced heart failure. J Heart Lung Transplant 2009;28(6):537.

United States is estimated to affect 250,000 to 500,000 people.[13]

NATURAL HISTORY

The clinical course of heart failure is progressive but nonlinear, characterized by worsening quality of life despite increasing levels of care[14] (**Fig. 2**). Early in the syndrome, the diagnosis of heart failure is established, and there is a period of initiation and titration of evidence-based pharmacologic and, when appropriate, implantation of electrical therapies to prevent sudden death and resynchronize ventricular contraction. Following this stage, there is often improvement leading to a stage of stability lasting months to years. However, as the disease progresses, functional status declines, resulting in multiple admissions for heart failure, which originally responds to therapy but ultimately becomes advanced and refractory to treatment. Once this occurs, only a few treatment options remain: ongoing supportive medical management, palliative inotropes, or consideration for advanced therapies including mechanical circulatory support (MCS) and transplantation.[14] The natural history of advanced heart failure is ultimately defined by the therapies deployed to combat this complex disease phenotype.

Systolic heart failure patients managed medically with angiotensin converting enzyme (ACE)-inhibitors, beta-adrenergic blockers, and mineralicorticoid receptor antagonists have experienced decreased mortality rates by 17%, 34%, and 30% respectively.[15] Even when these evidence-based pharmacotherapies are attempted, the natural course of advanced heart failure is dismal. This is best illustrated in the medical management arm of the REMATCH (Randomized Evaluation of Mechanical Assistance for the Treatment of Congestive Heart Failure) trial. This trial randomized patients with chronic systolic heart failure who were ineligible for transplantation to a pulsatile left ventricular assist device or optimum medical therapy. The aggregate survival of the medical arm at 1 and 2 years was 25% and 8%, respectively, with a median survival of only 150 days. The majority of patients within the medical therapy group died of progressive left ventricular dysfunction (93%) despite frequent inotrope use,[16] with few patients experiencing ventricular arrhythmias.

Multiple studies have examined the use of inotropes in patients with advanced heart failure. Frequently deployed in patients with relative hypotension and reduced ejection fraction, inotropes improve myocardial contractility and performance at the expense of increased myocardial oxygen consumption and arrhythmia risk. For example, the PROMISE trial (Randomized Milrinone Survival Evaluation), which randomized 1088 patients with advanced heart failure to oral milrinone or placebo, was stopped early due to a 28% increase in all-cause mortality and 34% increase in cardiovascular mortality in the oral milrinone group. Those patients identified as having the most severe heart failure (NYHA class 4 and low serum sodium) had significant increases in mortality.[17] In a more recent study, the inotrope arm of the INTrEPID trial (Chronic Mechanical Circulatory Support for Inotrope-Dependent Heart Failure Patients Who Are Not Transplant Candidates) showed a survival of 22% at 6 months and 11% at 1 year.[18] Despite the attendant risks, patients on inotropes often experience relief of dyspnea, improved end-organ function and a modestly improved functional capacity, requiring physicians and patients to consider trading length of life for improved quality.

Given the poor natural course of patients with advanced heart disease despite optimal oral medical therapy or inotropes, treatment with left ventricular assist devices (LVADs) or cardiac transplantation is attractive. Advanced surgical heart failure therapies have excellent long-term outcomes in select patients, but are limited by the number of donor hearts, considerable costs, and competing mortality risk from comorbid medical conditions. Mechanical circulatory support has recently become the most commonly used surgical therapy for advanced heart failure and is now uncoupled from transplant candidacy.[16] With the advent of continuous flow devices, the

Table 2
Definition of advanced heart failure across cardiovascular professional societies

	Refractory Symptoms					Exercise Intolerance	Objective Evidence of Severe Cardiac Dysfunction			
	Severe Symptoms	Multiple Hospitalizations	Optimal Therapy	Inotropic Support	Fluid Retention and/or Peripheral Hypoperfusion	Severe Functional Capacity Impairment	Reduced Ejection Fraction	Doppler Echocardiography	Hemodynamics	Elevated Natriuretic Peptides
ACC/AHA	x	x	x	—	—	x	x	—	—	—
HFSA	x	x	x	x	—	x	—	—	—	—
ESC	x	x	x	—	x	x	x	x	—	x

Abbreviations: ACC/AHA, American College of Cardiology/American Heart Association; ESC, European Society of Cardiology; HFSA, Heart Failure Society of America.
Adapted from Abouezzeddine OF, Redfield MM. Who has advanced heart failure?: definition and epidemiology. Congest Heart Fail 2011;17:162; with permission.

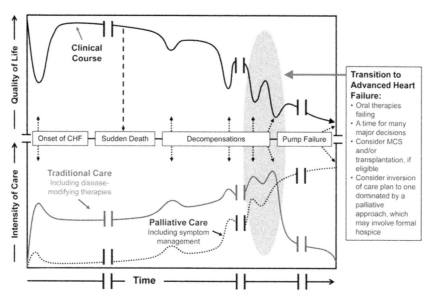

Fig. 2. Natural history of heart failure. This depiction of the clinical course of heart failure highlights the progressive, nonlinear course of disease marked by declining quality of life coupled with increasing care intensity that accelerates after the transition to advanced heart failure. CHF, chronic heart failure; MCS, mechanical circulatory support. (*From* Allen LA, Stevenson LW, Grady KL, et al. Decision making in advanced heart failure: a scientific statement from the American Heart Association. Circulation 2012;125(5):1930.)

1-year survival of patients with LVADs is now in excess of 80%.[19] Younger patients with advanced heart disease with fewer comorbid medical conditions who are fortunate enough to receive a transplant still have the best long-term course. Contemporary survival rates after heart transplantation are between 85% and 90% at 1 year, and median survival is 11 years for all and over 13 years for those surviving the first year.[20]

PROGNOSIS

Once advanced heart failure is suspected, recognition of those factors that may portend the poorest prognosis is important to target patients for early referral for evaluation of candidacy for advanced therapies or consolidation of palliation (**Box 1**). Important prognostic factors can be categorized broadly into 4 groups: clinical factors, the right heart, laboratory assessment, and medication intolerances.

Clinical Factors

A thorough history and physical examination are the first steps in assessing a patient with advanced heart failure, beginning with demographics. An analysis of the CHARM (Candesartan in Heart Failure and Reduction in Mortality and Morbidity) trial suggested all-cause mortality more than doubles with increasing age, with the largest increase in patients older than 70 years

of age.[21] A meta-analysis of 5 trials also revealed that, after adjustment for other known predictors of mortality, females had a 23% lower 1 year mortality rate than men for reasons that remain unclear.[22] Physical examination findings associated with advanced heart failure include resting tachycardia, narrow pulse pressure, hypotension, peripheral vasoconstriction, cardiac cachexia, and an audible S3 gallop.

A patient's NYHA class, an easily obtained, noninvasive evaluation of functional capacity, provides further prognostic information. Prior to the use of ACE inhibitors, a direct relationship between NYHA class and mortality had been consistently demonstrated, with 1 year mortality rates of patients with NYHA class 1, 2/3, or 4 of 5%, 15%, and 64%, respectively, even with contemporary neurohormonal therapy.[9,23–25] Other more objective evaluations of functional capacity such as cardiopulmonary exercise testing with oxygen uptake or 6-minute walk are also used to define prognosis. Patients with peak oxygen consumption of less than 10 to 12 mL/kg/min (or ≤50%–55% predicted) have superior outcomes with treatments such as mechanical circulatory support or transplant in comparison with on-going medical therapies.[10,26,27] However, many patients with advanced heart disease are unable to achieve adequate levels of effort required for the interpretation of peak oxygen consumption. For such patients, a minute ventilation–carbon dioxide production relationship

(VE/VCO2 slope) greater than 34 has been associated with poor prognosis.[28,29]

Careful review of a patient's recent clinical course can help predict the likelihood of morbidity and mortality. Solomon and colleagues[30] examined the CHARM database and showed a greater than 300% increase in mortality in patients discharged from the hospital after their first heart failure hospitalization. Subsequently, Setoguchi and colleagues[31] not only reconfirmed these findings but also showed an ongoing increase in mortality risk following each additional hospitalization even after adjustment for age and renal function (**Fig. 3**). The association between recurrent heart failure hospitalization and mortality represents progressive symptomatic decompensation as heart failure approaches its end stages.

Additional findings such as frailty, sarcopenia, and cachexia are emerging integrative markers of advanced cardiac disease. Frailty, defined as a decline in overall function and loss of resistance to stressors[32] can be diagnosed when a patient has unintentional weight loss, physical exhaustion by self-report, weakness by grip strength, decline in walking speed, and low physical activity.[10,33] Cacciatore and colleagues[34] were the first to demonstrate the relationship between frailty and mortality in patients with heart failure, noting a 24% increase in mortality when comparing the most frail to least frail patients in 12-year follow-up. The assessment of frailty prior to advanced therapies such as left ventricular assist device (LVAD) has now become routine.[35]

Cachexia and sarcopenia are thought to be part of a wasting continuum of the frailty syndrome seen in patients with advanced heart failure,[36] occurring secondary to a catabolic state caused by a combination of increased inflammatory cytokines, decreased testosterone levels, and increased insulin resistance.[37] Cachexia, defined as a loss of muscle and fat tissue resulting in weight loss, is noted in 10% to 15% of patients with heart failure and portends an extremely poor prognosis. Patients who developed cardiac cachexia (defined as a nonintentional weight loss of >7.5%) have nearly a fourfold increase of mortality at 18 months, independent of other known risk factors.[38] There also appears to be a direct relationship between degree of cachexia and mortality. In the subset of patients with the lowest degree of cachexia (defined as loss of 5% of body weight), there was a 1.4 fold increased risk of mortality, while those with the highest degree of cachexia (>15% of body weight) had a striking 3.3-fold increase in mortality.[39] Sarcopenia, which is characterized by a loss of skeletal muscle mass and strength that predominantly affects postural rather than nonpostural muscles, occurs in 20% of patients with heart failure. Although assumed to be a poor prognostic sign, the true implications of the presence of sarcopenia are undergoing active investigation.

Right Heart Factors

Once thought of as a passive conduit to the left ventricle, the importance of right ventricular function in the prognosis of patients with advanced heart failure is now well recognized. Right heart failure and associated pulmonary hypertension can occur by multiple processes:

- An increase in right ventricular afterload due to left ventricular failure

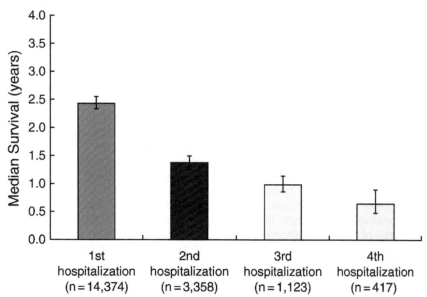

Fig. 3. Impact of recurrent heart failure hospitalization on mortality. Median survival (50% mortality) with 95% confidence limits in patients with heart failure after each heart failure hospitalization. (*From* Setoguchi S, Stevenson LW, Schneeweiss S. Repeated hospitalizations predict mortality in the community population with heart failure. Am Heart J 2007;154(2):262; with permission.)

- An intrinsic cardiomyopathic process or prior injury
- Decreased systolic driving pressure of the right ventricular coronary perfusion
- Ventricular interdependence due to septal dysfunction/bowing[40]

In patients with advanced heart failure, right ventricular ejection fraction of at least 35% has been consistently demonstrated to be a potent predictor of survival, and may be even more important than peak oxygen consumption.[41] Right heart function is load dependent, so studies have also focused on pulmonary pressures. Mortality in dilated cardiomyopathy has been shown to increase 25% for every 5 mm Hg in mean pulmonary pressure, with pulmonary vascular resistance increased above 3 Wood units conferring an 86% increased risk of death.[42] Right heart failure may also be an important mediator of the metabolic derangements contributing to cardiac cachexia and sarcopenia. Early recognition and treatment of right heart failure and pulmonary hypertension is important in patients with advanced heart failure and may influence eligibility for advanced mechanical support or cardiac transplantation.

Laboratory Assessment

Progressive cardiac failure is characterized by neurohormonal dysregulation leading to a series of pathophysiologic derangements readily assayed with routine blood tests. Various laboratory abnormalities are associated with poor prognosis, with the 2 most ominous being hyponatremia and worsening renal function (cardiorenal syndrome). Hyponatremia results from increased levels of norepinephrine, renin, and ADH through multiple mechanisms: increase in water reabsorption in the collecting tubules of the nephron, limitation of water excretion, and stimulation of thirst.[43,44] Although commonly noted among patients with advanced heart failure, the true prevalence is unknown given the lack of a standardized definition in the literature. In an older study by Lee and Packer,[45] low serum sodium concentration (Na < 137) was the most powerful predictor of long-term prognosis. The link between hyponatremia and increased mortality appears to be maintained regardless of ejection fraction, although it portends a worse prognosis in the patients with HFrEF.[46] Other independent markers of risk in advanced heart failure include hyperuricemia, anemia, and hypoalbuminemia.

The cardiorenal syndrome is common in advanced heart failure and arises when attempts to relieve congestion are limited by worsening renal function.[47] More than 60% of patients admitted to the hospital with acute heart failure may demonstrate this syndrome,[10] related to a combination of neurohormonal adaptations, reduced renal perfusion, increased renal venous pressure, and right ventricular dysfunction.[47] A meta-analysis of 16 studies showed increasing mortality rates of 24%, 38%, and 51%, with greater degrees of renal dysfunction (glomerular filtration rate [GFR] > 90, GFR 53–89, and GFR <53 mL/min respectively).[48] The cardiorenal syndrome can also impact outcomes after mechanical support for advanced heart failure. A recent INTERMACS study demonstrated a 20% reduction in survival in patients with the worst compared to best degree of renal function.[49]

The circulating natriuretic peptides, B-type natriuretic peptide (BNP) and its prohormone NT-proBNP, are secreted by the heart chambers in response to increased wall stress and have become prognostic biomarkers for heart failure. A systematic review of 19 trials showed a 35% increase in the relative risk of death for every 100 pg/mL increase of BNP.[50] Additionally, survival in patients who are able to normalize their BNP levels after 3 months of optimal medical therapy is nearly 3.5 times higher than those who cannot.[51] However, in the subset of patients with advanced heart failure, natriuretic peptide levels can be more labile and have been less robustly associated with outcomes. Natriutetic peptide levels should only be used in conjunction with additional prognostic factors in this cohort of patients. Other biomarkers of cardiac remodeling such as ST-2 and galectin-3, markers of cardiac stress and fibrosis, are frequently abnormal in systolic heart failure but have not yet been shown to have a robust independent role in the care of patients with advanced disease.

Medication Intolerance

The standard of care for medical management in patients with advanced heart failure includes diuretics, ACE inhibitors, beta-blockers, and aldosterone receptor antagonists. Although sacubatril–valsartan is approved for use in patients with NYHA class 4 heart failure with reduced ejection fraction, data on its optimal dosing safety and effectiveness remain limited. Many patients with stage D heart failure cannot tolerate the target doses of those neurohormonal agents proven to have mortality benefit in pivotal trials. Patients intolerant of guideline-directed heart failure therapies or those who require progressively lower doses have been convincingly shown to have worse prognosis.

Up to one-third of advanced heart failure patients admitted to the hospital may be unable to be discharged on an ACE inhibitor predominantly because of circulatory–renal complications such as renal insufficiency or symptomatic hypotension.[52] Those patients unable to tolerate ACE inhibition have a 2.5-fold higher incidence of death, ventricular assist device placement, and transplantation. Similarly, the inability to tolerate

beta-blockade due to hypotension, bradycardia, or fatigue has also been associated with poor prognosis.[52] Patients discharged without a beta-blocker had nearly double the mortality of those discharged on beta-blockade.[53]

Diuretic resistance is defined as the progressive increase in diuretic dose required to achieve net fluid balanced and has been attributed to pump failure, hyperaldosteronism, or dietary indiscretion. A retrospective evaluation of the PRAISE (Prospective Randomized Amlodipine Survival and Evaluation) trial suggested a progressive increase in mortality based on the quartile of diuretic dose prescribed (21% in lowest quartile, 45% in highest quartile). Additionally, the use of metolazone was also shown to be an independent predictor of mortality in this subset of patients.[54] It is not yet known if the increase in mortality is secondary to drug effect or is an independent marker of worsened heart failure.[55]

Multimarker models such as the Seattle Heart Failure Score (SHFS) and Heart Failure Survival Score (HFSS) have been used to integrate prognostic markers into a single score to better identify the subset of patients most likely to benefit from urgent evaluation for transplantation or mechanical circulatory support. However, these models include data derived from populations of younger patients with mild-to-moderate heart failure[56] and prior to modern advances such as cardiac resynchronization therapy,[57] resulting in poorly calibrated estimates of mortality once advanced disease is present.[58] Given the high degree of prognostic uncertainty and the complex trade-offs required to select between different treatment options, a thoughtful approach to communication with patients is required. Proactive patient engagement and serial education about prognosis at an annual heart failure review can lay the foundation for shared decisions in this complex syndrome.[14]

SUMMARY

Advanced heart failure is an epidemic estimated to affect approximately 5% of the general population with heart failure. Understanding the natural history and prognostic signs associated with transition to advanced disease is required for timely evaluation for advanced therapies or end-of-life palliative treatments that are consistent with a patient's values, preferences, and goals. Additional articles in this issue of *Heart Failure Clinics* will focus on the interaction between the failing heart and end–organ function, the biologic basis of advanced heart failure, and the evolving role of advanced medical, electrical, and surgical therapies.

REFERENCES

1. Yancy CW, Jessup M, Bozkurt B, et al. 2013 ACCF/AHA guideline for the management of heart failure: executive summary: a report of the American College of Cardiology Foundation/American Heart Association Task Force on practice guidelines. Circulation 2013;128(16):1810–52.

2. Bui AL, Horwich TB, Fonarow GC. Epidemiology and risk profile of heart failure. Nat Rev Cardiol 2011; 8(1):30–41.

3. Mozaffarian D, Benjamin EJ, Go AS, et al. Heart disease and stroke statistics–2016 update: a report from the American Heart Association. Circulation 2016;133(4):e38–360.

4. Heart Failure Society of America, Lindenfeld J, Albert NM, et al. HFSA 2010 comprehensive heart failure practice guideline. J Card Fail 2010;16(6): e1–194.

5. McMurray JJ, Adamopoulos S, Anker SD, et al. ESC guidelines for the diagnosis and treatment of acute and chronic heart failure 2012: the task force for the diagnosis and treatment of acute and chronic heart failure 2012 of the European Society of Cardiology. Developed in collaboration with the Heart Failure Association (HFA) of the ESC. Eur Heart J 2012; 33(14):1787–847.

6. The criteria committee of the New York Heart Association. Nomenclature and criteria for diagnosis of diseases of the heart and great vessels. 9th edition. Boston: Little, Brown, Co; 1994. p. 253.

7. Stevenson LW, Pagani FD, Young JB, et al. INTERMACS profiles of advanced heart failure: the current picture. J Heart Lung Transplant 2009;28(6):535–41.

8. Abouezzeddine OF, Redfield MM. Who has advanced heart failure?: definition and epidemiology. Congest Heart Fail 2011;17(4):160–8.

9. Group TCTS. Effects of enalapril on mortality in severe congestive heart failure. Results of the Cooperative North Scandinavian Enalapril Survival Study (CONSENSUS). The CONSENSUS Trial Study Group. N Engl J Med 1987;316(23):1429–35.

10. Fang JC, Ewald GA, Allen LA, et al. Advanced (stage D) heart failure: a statement from the heart failure society of America guidelines committee. J Card Fail 2015;21(6):519–34.

11. Ammar KA, Jacobsen SJ, Mahoney DW, et al. Prevalence and prognostic significance of heart failure stages: application of the American College of Cardiology/American Heart Association heart failure staging criteria in the community. Circulation 2007; 115(12):1563–70.

12. Costanzo MR, Mills RM, Wynne J. Characteristics of "Stage D" heart failure: insights from the acute decompensated heart failure national registry longitudinal module (ADHERE LM). Am Heart J 2008; 155(2):339–47.

13. Norton C, Georgiopoulou VV, Kalogeropoulos AP, et al. Epidemiology and cost of advanced heart failure. Prog Cardiovasc Dis 2011;54(2):78–85.

14. Allen LA, Stevenson LW, Grady KL, et al. Decision making in advanced heart failure: a scientific statement from the American Heart Association. Circulation 2012;125(15):1928–52.

15. Fonarow GC, Yancy CW, Hernandez AF, et al. Potential impact of optimal implementation of evidence-based heart failure therapies on mortality. Am Heart J 2011;161(6):1024–30.e3.

16. Rose EA, Gelijns AC, Moskowitz AJ, et al. Long-term use of a left ventricular assist device for end-stage heart failure. N Engl J Med 2001;345(20):1435–43.

17. Packer M, Carver JR, Rodeheffer RJ, et al. Effect of oral milrinone on mortality in severe chronic heart failure. The PROMISE Study Research Group. N Engl J Med 1991;325(21):1468–75.

18. Rogers JG, Butler J, Lansman SL, et al. Chronic mechanical circulatory support for inotrope-dependent heart failure patients who are not transplant candidates: results of the INTrEPID Trial. J Am Coll Cardiol 2007;50(8):741–7.

19. Kirklin JK, Naftel DC, Pagani FD, et al. Sixth INTERMACS annual report: a 10,000-patient database. J Heart Lung Transplant 2014;33(6):555–64.

20. Lund LH, Edwards LB, Kucheryavaya AY, et al. The registry of the international society for heart and lung transplantation: thirty-second official adult heart transplantation report–2015; focus theme: early graft failure. J Heart Lung Transplant 2015; 34(10):1244–54.

21. Wong CM, Hawkins NM, Jhund PS, et al. Clinical characteristics and outcomes of young and very young adults with heart failure: the CHARM programme (candesartan in heart failure assessment of reduction in mortality and morbidity). J Am Coll Cardiol 2013;62(20):1845–54.

22. Frazier CG, Alexander KP, Newby LK, et al. Associations of gender and etiology with outcomes in heart failure with systolic dysfunction: a pooled analysis of 5 randomized control trials. J Am Coll Cardiol 2007; 49(13):1450–8.

23. Effect of enalapril on mortality and the development of heart failure in asymptomatic patients with reduced left ventricular ejection fractions. The SOLVD Investigattors. N Engl J Med 1992;327(10): 685–91.

24. Effect of enalapril on survival in patients with reduced left ventricular ejection fractions and congestive heart failure. The SOLVD Investigators. N Engl J Med 1991;325(5):293–302.

25. Greenberg B, Lottes SR, Nelson JJ, et al. Predictors of clinical outcomes in patients given carvedilol for heart failure. Am J Cardiol 2006;98(11):1480–4.

26. Mancini DM, Eisen H, Kussmaul W, et al. Value of peak exercise oxygen consumption for optimal timing

of cardiac transplantation in ambulatory patients with heart failure. Circulation 1991;83(3):778–86.

27. Peterson LR, Schechtman KB, Ewald GA, et al. Timing of cardiac transplantation in patients with heart failure receiving beta-adrenergic blockers. J Heart Lung Transplant 2003;22(10):1141–8.

28. Chua TP, Ponikowski P, Harrington D, et al. Clinical correlates and prognostic significance of the ventilatory response to exercise in chronic heart failure. J Am Coll Cardiol 1997;29(7):1585–90.

29. Balady GJ, Arena R, Sietsema K, et al. Clinician's guide to cardiopulmonary exercise testing in adults: a scientific statement from the American Heart Association. Circulation 2010;122(2):191–225.

30. Solomon SD, Dobson J, Pocock S, et al. Influence of nonfatal hospitalization for heart failure on subsequent mortality in patients with chronic heart failure. Circulation 2007;116(13):1482–7.

31. Setoguchi S, Stevenson LW, Schneeweiss S. Repeated hospitalizations predict mortality in the community population with heart failure. Am Heart J 2007;154(2):260–6.

32. McNallan SM, Chamberlain AM, Gerber Y, et al. Measuring frailty in heart failure: a community perspective. Am Heart J 2013;166(4):768–74.

33. Fried LP, Tangen CM, Walston J, et al. Frailty in older adults: evidence for a phenotype. J Gerontol A Biol Sci Med Sci 2001;56(3):M146–56.

34. Cacciatore F, Abete P, Mazzella F, et al. Frailty predicts long-term mortality in elderly subjects with chronic heart failure. Eur J Clin Invest 2005;35(12):723–30.

35. Flint KM, Matlock DD, Lindenfeld J, et al. Frailty and the selection of patients for destination therapy left ventricular assist device. Circ Heart Fail 2012;5(2):286–93.

36. Von Haehling S. The wasting continuum in heart failure: from sarcopenia to cachexia. Proc Nutr Soc 2015;74:367–77.

37. Afilalo J, Alexander KP, Mack MJ, et al. Frailty assessment in the cardiovascular care of older adults. J Am Coll Cardiol 2014;63(8):747–62.

38. Anker SD, Ponikowski P, Varney S, et al. Wasting as independent risk factor for mortality in chronic heart failure. Lancet 1997;349(9058):1050–3.

39. Anker SD, Negassa A, Coats AJ, et al. Prognostic importance of weight loss in chronic heart failure and the effect of treatment with angiotensin-converting-enzyme inhibitors: an observational study. Lancet 2003;361(9363):1077–83.

40. Voelkel NF, Quaife RA, Leinwand LA, et al. Right ventricular function and failure: report of a National Heart, Lung, and Blood Institute working group on cellular and molecular mechanisms of right heart failure. Circulation 2006;114(17):1883–91.

41. Di Salvo TG, Mathier M, Semigran MJ, et al. Preserved right ventricular ejection fraction predicts

42. Cappola TP, Felker GM, Kao WH, et al. Pulmonary hypertension and risk of death in cardiomyopathy: patients with myocarditis are at higher risk. Circulation 2002;105(14):1663–8.

43. Verbrugge FH, Steels P, Grieten L, et al. Hyponatremia in acute decompensated heart failure: depletion versus dilution. J Am Coll Cardiol 2015;65(5):480–92.

44. Kumar S, Rubin S, Mather PJ, et al. Hyponatremia and vasopressin antagonism in congestive heart failure. Clin Cardiol 2007;30(11):546–51.

45. Lee WH, Packer M. Prognostic importance of serum sodium concentration and its modification by converting-enzyme inhibition in patients with severe chronic heart failure. Circulation 1986;73(2):257–67.

46. Rusinaru D, Tribouilloy C, Berry C, et al. Relationship of serum sodium concentration to mortality in a wide spectrum of heart failure patients with preserved and with reduced ejection fraction: an individual patient data meta-analysis(dagger): meta-analysis global group in chronic heart failure (MAGGIC). Eur J Heart Fail 2012;14(10):1139–46.

47. Bock JS, Gottlieb SS. Cardiorenal syndrome: new perspectives. Circulation 2010;121(23):2592–600.

48. Smith GL, Lichtman JH, Bracken MB, et al. Renal impairment and outcomes in heart failure: systematic review and meta-analysis. J Am Coll Cardiol 2006;47(10):1987–96.

49. Kirklin JK, Naftel DC, Kormos RL, et al. Quantifying the effect of cardiorenal syndrome on mortality after left ventricular assist device implant. J Heart Lung Transplant 2013;32(12):1205–13.

50. Doust JA, Pietrzak E, Dobson A, et al. How well does B-type natriuretic peptide predict death and cardiac events in patients with heart failure: systematic review. BMJ 2005;330(7492):625.

51. Maeda K, Tsutamoto T, Wada A, et al. High levels of plasma brain natriuretic peptide and interleukin-6 after optimized treatment for heart failure are independent risk factors for morbidity and mortality in patients with congestive heart failure. J Am Coll Cardiol 2000;36(5):1587–93.

52. Kittleson M, Hurwitz S, Shah MR, et al. Development of circulatory-renal limitations to angiotensin-converting enzyme inhibitors identifies patients with severe heart failure and early mortality. J Am Coll Cardiol 2003;41(11):2029–35.

53. Fonarow GC, Abraham WT, Albert NM, et al. Prospective evaluation of beta-blocker use at the time of hospital discharge as a heart failure performance measure: results from OPTIMIZE-HF. J Card Fail 2007;13(9):722–31.

54. Neuberg GW, Miller AB, O'Connor CM, et al. Diuretic resistance predicts mortality in patients

exercise capacity and survival in advanced heart failure. J Am Coll Cardiol 1995;25(5):1143–53.

with advanced heart failure. Am Heart J 2002; 144(1):31–8.

55. Mielniczuk LM, Tsang SW, Desai AS, et al. The association between high-dose diuretics and clinical stability in ambulatory chronic heart failure patients. J Card Fail 2008;14(5):388–93.

56. Levy WC, Mozaffarian D, Linker DT, et al. The Seattle heart failure model: prediction of survival in heart failure. Circulation 2006;113(11):1424–33.

57. Aaronson KD, Schwartz JS, Chen TM, et al. Development and prospective validation of a clinical index to predict survival in ambulatory patients referred for cardiac transplant evaluation. Circulation 1997; 95(12):2660–7.

58. Gorodeski EZ, Chu EC, Chow CH, et al. Application of the Seattle heart failure model in ambulatory patients presented to an advanced heart failure therapeutics committee. Circ Heart Fail 2010;3(6):706–14.

Cardiorenal Interactions

Valentina Carubelli, MD[a], Carlo Lombardi, MD[a],*, Elio Gorga, MD[a],
Alice Ravera, MD[a], Marco Metra, MD[a], Robert J. Mentz, MD[b]

KEYWORDS

- Heart failure • Acute heart failure • Renal dysfunction • Worsening renal function
- Renal biomarkers • Chronic kidney disease

KEY POINTS

- The prevalence of comorbidities, including renal dysfunction, is high and growing in patients with heart failure.
- Renal dysfunction is associated with suboptimal treatment response and worse outcomes in heart failure patients.
- Early identification of renal damage and targeted therapy could avoid the progression of the cardiorenal syndrome.
- New renal biomarkers may allow for earlier detection of acute kidney injury compared with current routine laboratory values and many of these have been associated with outcomes in patients with heart failure.
- The treatment of cardiorenal syndrome requires a tailored approach based on a patient's underlying pathophysiology. Several new approaches and novel drugs seem promising.

INTRODUCTION

Heart failure (HF) is a major public health problem affecting 1% to 2% of the adult population in developed countries.[1] In the United States, approximately 5 million persons have clinical HF with a prevalence that is expected to increase by 46% in the next several decades.[2,3] Although the development and implementation of novel therapies for patients with HF with reduced ejection fraction has improved survival in recent years, mortality rates remain unacceptably high, reaching 50% within 5 years of diagnosis.[3,4] The prognosis of patients hospitalized for acute HF (AHF) is even worse with high mortality and rehospitalization rates in the so-called vulnerable period after discharge.[5] HF hospitalization is the leading cause of admission in Western countries and is responsible for a large percentage of the financial burden of this disease.[6] Importantly, the overall aging of

the population is an important reason for the growing HF prevalence worldwide.[7] Notably, elderly patients are frequently affected by noncardiac comorbidities that contribute to further progression of the primary disease and complicate disease management. Comorbidities are associated with an attenuated response to HF treatment and worse clinical outcomes.[8] Epidemiological studies show that between 1988 and 2008 the proportion of US patients older than 80 years increased from 13.3% to 22.4% with a concomitant increase in patients with 5 or more comorbidities from 42% to 58%.[9]

Among comorbidities, renal dysfunction is one of the most common conditions in the HF setting.[8] Indeed, cardiac and renal functions are closely linked, and the term cardiorenal syndrome (CRS) has been introduced in recent years to characterize this interaction. Patients with HF may develop different degrees of renal dysfunction

[a] Cardiology, Department of Medical and Surgical Specialties, Radiological Sciences and Public Health, University of Brescia, P.zza Spedali Civili 1, Brescia 25123, Italy; [b] Duke University Medical Center, Duke Clinical Research Institute, Pratt Street, Durham, NC 27705, USA
* Corresponding author. P.zza Spedali Civili 1, Brescia 25123, Italy.
E-mail address: lombardi.carlo@alice.it

Heart Failure Clin 12 (2016) 335–347
http://dx.doi.org/10.1016/j.hfc.2016.03.002
1551-7136/16/$ – see front matter © 2016 Elsevier Inc. All rights reserved.

merely due to underlying HF, even in absence of a primary renal disease.[10] On the other hand, cardiovascular risk factors such as hypertension and diabetes are the leading cause of chronic kidney disease (CKD) in the general population, which is in turn associated with accelerated atherosclerosis and cardiovascular events, including the development and exacerbation of underlying HF.[11] The treatment of HF, specifically the use of diuretics, may further contribute to the decline of renal function, especially in the acute phase. Worsening renal function (WRF), defined as an increase of serum creatinine (sCr) greater than or equal to 0.3 mg/dL, has been recognized as an important negative prognostic predictor in hospitalized patients.[12] Renal dysfunction is associated with suboptimal treatment response and worse outcomes in both acute and chronic HF patients.[12–15]

The high prevalence and adverse associations between renal dysfunction and HF outcomes have led to a focus in both routine clinical practice and clinical investigation on the diagnosis and management of comorbid renal dysfunction. Several new biomarkers have been identified in recent years to better quantify and allow for earlier detection of declines in renal function.[16] Despite the investigative focus on CRS in recent years, and aside from neurohormonal blocking agents (eg, angiotensin-converting enzyme inhibitor/angiotensin receptor blockers), broadly applicable treatments for CRS in HF patients are lacking. However, preliminary data support several novel therapies. This article summarizes the current understanding of cardiorenal interactions, focusing on the usefulness of markers of kidney damage and on the effects of treatment on kidney function.

HEART FAILURE AND RENAL FUNCTION
Epidemiology

Renal dysfunction is a significant independent predictor of rehospitalization and mortality in patients with HF.[17] Among patients with chronic stable HF,

the prevalence of CKD is up to 30%.[18,19] In patients with AHF, the prevalence of renal dysfunction is approximately 30% to 60%, depending on the specific definition.[20–22] Furthermore, in-hospital WRF is a common complication during HF hospitalization and an independent predictor of long-term mortality in previous studies.[23–25] However, recent evidence has suggested conflicting data about the association between changes in creatinine and prognosis. In the Diuretic Optimization Strategies Evaluation (DOSE) trial, it was observed that subjects who were treated with high diuretic doses had a greater deterioration of renal function but this did not affect outcomes.[26] Other studies have also demonstrated that WRF may be a transient epiphenomenon related to effective decongestion.[27] In this context, the value of sCr changes in predicting acute kidney injury (AKI) should be reconsidered.

Cardiorenal Syndrome

CRS is a term commonly used to describe a clinical situation in which renal dysfunction and cardiac dysfunction coexist.[28] Multiple mechanisms may be involved in the development of CRS (**Table 1**). The heart and kidney interact bidirectionally. The mechanisms leading to renal dysfunction in patients with HF include congestion, hemodynamic alterations, neurohormonal and inflammatory activation and also release of adenosine and arginine-vasopressin (AVP) (**Fig. 1**).[29] Recently, the roles of anemia and iron deficiency have been underscored as fundamental components in the pathophysiology of CRS. Thus, the term cardio-renal anemia syndrome has been introduced.[30]

HOW TO ASSESS RENAL DYSFUNCTION
Serum Creatinine, Glomerular Filtration Rate, and Blood Urea Nitrogen

sCr and glomerular filtration rate (GFR) remain the cornerstone diagnostic tests evaluation of renal

Table 1
Consensus Conference of Acute Dialysis Quality Initiative Group classification of cardiorenal syndromes

Type	Pathophysiology	Consequences
Type 1	Acute worsening of heart function	Kidney injury and/or dysfunction
Type 2	Chronic abnormalities in heart function	Kidney injury and/or dysfunction
Type 3	Acute worsening of kidney function or AKI	Heart injury and/or dysfunction
Type 4	CKD	Heart injury and/or dysfunction
Type 5	Systemic conditions	Simultaneous injury and/or dysfunction of heart and kidney

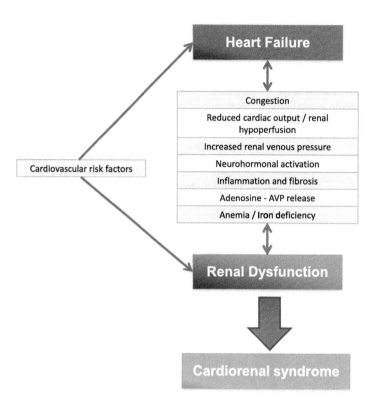

Fig. 1. Pathophysiological mechanisms of CRS.

function due to their wide availability. According to the National Kidney Foundation Kidney Disease Outcomes Quality Initiative (K/DOQI) Guidelines, the staging of CKD is defined by GFR values.[31] In clinical practice, estimated GFR (eGFR) uses formulas such as those from the Chronic Kidney Disease Epidemiology Collaboration (CKD-EPI) and/or the Modification of Diet in Renal Disease (MDRD).[32,33] However, sCr and, consequently, eGFR based on sCr value are far from optimal renal function markers (**Table 2**). The sCr concentration is influenced by age, gender, and muscle mass.[20] This is a critical issue in patients with advanced HF who have muscle loss due to a hypercatabolic state, leading to a significant underestimation of renal dysfunction. Another issue with sCr is related to the nonlinear relationship with GFR, given that modest increases in sCr may reflect a significant deterioration of GFR in patients with normal or mildly reduced renal function.[34] Beyond these limitations, sCr has slow kinetics that lead to delayed detection of AKI, especially in patients with severe renal dysfunction.[35]

To address several of these considerations, the evaluation of AKI in clinical practice is currently based on both sCr and GFR, in addition to urine output using the classifications Risk of renal failure, Injury to the kidney, Failure of the kidney, Loss of kidney function, and End-stage kidney disease (RIFLE) and the Acute Kidney Injury Network (AKIN).[36,37]

Another marker widely used in clinical practice to characterize renal dysfunction is blood urea nitrogen (BUN). In contrast to sCr, urea is reabsorbed by an AVP-mediated system in the collecting ducts, thus contributing to the regulation of the volume status. In conditions of AVP overexpression such as the underfilling state due to intensive diuretic treatment, urea is highly reabsorbed, increasing its blood concentration. In this situation, BUN may represent a useful marker of over-diuresis and can help to guide diuretic therapy. In conditions of low cardiac output, the increased renin-angiotensin aldosterone system (RAAS) and adrenergic stimulation lead to enhanced fluid and sodium retention. Consequently, distal tubule flow is reduced and there is increased urea reabsorption.[38] This important link between BUN and neurohormonal activation may at least partially explain the strong prognostic role of BUN in patients with acute or chronic HF. Indeed, in a second analysis of PROTECT, BUN was the strongest predictor of early events.[39] In the chronic HF setting, baseline BUN and changes over time have been associated with long-term clinical outcomes.[40]

Table 2
Old and novel renal biomarkers

Biomarker	Type	Advantages	Disadvantages	Relationship with Outcomes in HF
sCr	Renal function	Wide availability High clinical applicability	Influenced by age, gender, and muscle mass Nonlinear relationship with GFR Slow kinetics Delayed detection of AKI Not specific for renal tubular damage	Associated with prognosis in both acute and chronic HF In AHF setting, small increases may have negative prognostic significance only during deterioration of clinical status
GFR	Renal function	Wide availability Easily estimated	Dosing requires 24 h urine collection Estimation has possible bias (eg, elderly, extreme values)	Associated with prognosis in both acute and chronic HF In AHF setting, decreases may have negative prognostic significance only during deterioration of clinical status
BUN	Renal function Tubular function Neurohormonal activation Protein metabolism	Wide availability Early detection of underfilling condition	Influenced by protein hypercatabolism and nutritional status	Strong association with outcomes in both acute and chronic HF
CysC	Renal function (serum CysC) Tubular function (urinary CysC)	Serum CysC reflects GFR better than creatinine Independent of the body mass, protein intake, or catabolism	Not widely available in clinical practice High cost Urinary CysC is still poorly studied in HF	Associated with prognosis in acute and chronic HF Poor association with WRF
NGAL	Tubular function	Early increase during AKI High sensitivity in detecting subclinical AKI in the absence of increases in sCr	Not widely available in clinical practice High cost Plasma NGAL is less specific, increasing also during chronic inflammatory conditions and infections	Associated with mortality in acute and chronic HF Less evidences are available regarding rehospitalization
KIM-1	Tubular function	Early marker of proximal tubular damage Early detection of AKI, especially in chronic HF	Measured only in urine Not widely available in clinical practice High cost	Prognostic significance in HF remains controversial
NAG	Tubular function	Early marker of proximal tubular	Less studied compared with	Associated with prognosis in

(continued on next page)

Table 2
(continued)

Biomarker	Type	Advantages	Disadvantages	Relationship with Outcomes in HF
		damage May predict the reduction of renal perfusion Concentrations correlates with NT-proBNP levels	other markers Possible false-positive results Not widely available in clinical practice	chronic HF Few data are available in AHF
Interleukin-18	Inflammation	Quickly upregulated in response to AKI	Overexpressed in many different inflammatory conditions Few studies in HF-subjects	Modest association with WRF.
FABPs	Tubular function	Marker of tubular and interstitial damage Urine levels correlated with urine protein and sCr levels Early detection of AKI	Few studies in HF subjects	H-FABP was associated with AKI and in-hospital mortality in AHF
Proenkephalin	Renal function	Rapid variations according to renal function	Lack of studies No studies in subjects with HF	No data in HF

Abbreviations: BUN, blood urea nitrogen; CysC, cystatin C; FABPs, fatty-acid binding proteins; H-FABP, heart-type fatty-acid binding protein; KIM-1, kidney injury molecule 1; NAG, N-acetyl-beta-D-glucosaminidase; NGAL, neutrophil gelatinase-associated lipocalin; NT-proBNP, N-terminal of the prohormone brain natriuretic petide.

From a metabolic point of view, BUN is the final product of protein degradation, necessary for nitrogen excretion.[38] Accordingly, BUN is increased during muscle-wasting conditions such as advanced HF in which there is a progressive mobilization of amino acids, resulting in muscle mass loss and cardiac cachexia. Thus, BUN characterizes volume status, renal dysfunction, RAAS activation, and protein metabolism.

Novel Biomarkers

Several new biomarkers of renal function have been evaluated for their prognostic utility in recent years (see **Table 2**). Cystatin C (CysC) is a protein freely filtered by the glomerulus and subsequently reabsorbed by the tubules where it is catabolized.[41] Serum CysC is a marker of renal and glomerular function, whereas urine CysC (not reabsorbed by tubules) is a tubular function marker.[16] Studies suggest that it may be a valuable biomarker that adds incremental insights related to renal function beyond creatinine, GFR,

and BUN.[42] CysC shows a strong correlation with renal function.[43] In patients with chronic HF, data suggest that CysC may offer incremental prognostic value compared with sCr.[44] In the Acute Study of Clinical Effectiveness of Nesiritide in Decompensated Heart Failure (ASCEND-HF) biomarker substudy, baseline CysC value was associated with 30-day events and 180-day mortality. However, WRF as characterized by increases in CysC levels was not predictive of outcomes.[45]

Another component of AKI is characterized by tubular cell damage that may result in long-term organ dysfunction. In this context, potentially informative markers measure renal injury rather than renal function. Neutrophil gelatinase-associated lipocalin (NGAL) is a tubular function marker, detectable in both blood and urine, that is released after ischemic or toxic damage. NGAL shows an early increase during AKI.[46] In HF patients, NGAL was associated with both sCr and GFR, demonstrating the presence of tubular damage in stable subjects.[47] In addition, a recent study suggested that NGAL may offer advantages compared with CysC in the early detection of AKI in patients hospitalized for AHF.[48]

Kidney injury molecule-1 (KIM-1) is a marker of proximal tubule injury and inflammation.[49] Multiple studies have demonstrated the sensitivity of urinary KIM-1 for early detection of AKI and its association with adverse outcomes in CKD.[50,51] Although previous studies have found an association between KIM-1 and outcomes, the prognostic significance of KIM-1 in HF remains controversial.[52,53] In the recent subanalysis of the ASCEND-HF trial, the investigators did not confirm previous data supporting the incremental prognostic value of KIM-1.[54] In another study, KIM-1 was not associated with mortality in either acute or chronic HF patients.[55]

N-acetyl-beta-D-glucosaminidase (NAG) is localized in lysosomes in the proximal tubule. NAG has been shown to be associated with AKI in several clinical settings.[50,56,57] NAG levels correlate with renal plasma flow, highlighting the potential utility for detecting the reduction of renal perfusion in patients with low cardiac output.[52] In chronic HF, NAG was a predictor of long-term outcomes in association with eGFR and albumin-to-creatinine ratio.[58] Another study confirmed the predictive value of NAG independent of other markers of renal function such as GFR.[52]

Inflammation plays a central role during AKI. Interleukin-18 (IL-18) is often highly expressed during AKI, preceding the increase of renal function biomarkers, but after tubular markers increase.[59] A small study in AHF showed that despite a poor correlation with AKI, urinary IL-18 was associated with all-cause mortality.[60] The major limitation of IL-18 is low specificity because it is overexpressed in many different inflammatory conditions.

Fatty acid–binding proteins (FABPs) comprise a family of 9 isoforms of cytoplasmic proteins. The liver-FABP (L-FABP) isoform is expressed in the proximal renal tubular cells and is protective against oxidative stress,[61] whereas the heart-FABP (H-FABP) isoform is located in both the distal tubules and in the myocardium. Urinary L-FABP has been shown to have prognostic utility for AKI after cardiac surgery and in intensive care unit patients.[62,63] In AHF, H-FABP was also a predictor of WRF.[64] Further studies of the potential prognostic utility of FABPs are warranted in HF patients.

Recently, the use of combined biomarkers or a multimarker approach has been proposed for the early detection of AKI.[65,66] Evidence from the postoperative period has shown improved prediction of AKI implementing urinary NGAL, KIM-1, and NAG compared with using a single-biomarker strategy.[67,68] Moreover, additional novel molecules that characterize CRS are currently under investigation, such as proenkephalin, which has been correlated with cardiorenal status in post-myocardial infarction patients.[69]

TREATMENT OF CARDIORENAL SYNDROME
Diuretics and Diuretic Response

Loop diuretics are the cornerstone of congestion management in the treatment of symptomatic HF[70] and, despite their widespread use in clinical practice, several challenges persist regarding how to optimize therapeutic strategies. The current treatment of congestion, mainly based on loop diuretics, is unsatisfactory because patients with advanced HF may have a poor response to diuretics and inadequate congestion relief.[71] The so-called diuretic resistance, defined as the failure to relieve congestion despite an escalating dose of diuretics, is an emerging issue in the treatment of CRS. Diuretic resistance leads to detrimental consequences on fluid and sodium balance, and, eventually, to progressive refractoriness to therapeutic interventions.[72] Diuretic response (DR) and effectiveness is usually evaluated based on urine output and weight change. Recently, additional measures of DR have been proposed.[73] A surrogate method to evaluate effective decongestion is hemoconcentration. In one study, subjects with hemoconcentration (defined by change in hematocrit, albumin, and total proteins), despite a transitory WRF due to diuretic treatment, were shown to have better prognosis compared with subjects without hemoconcentration.[74] Testani and colleagues[75] estimated DR as the net fluid output per 40 mg of furosemide and demonstrated that patients with low diuretic responsiveness had an increased risk of death. In this study, DR was poorly correlated with both urine output and furosemide dose, indicating that this variable carries incremental insights compared with its components. Another approach, proposed by Valente and colleagues,[76] involves the ratio between change of body weight for 40 mg of furosemide. In an analysis from the PROTECT trial, low DR by day 4 was observed in sicker patients and increased both mortality and HF rehospitalization. Subsequent studies confirmed these findings.[77,78] However, a recent study raised some concerns about the reliability of these metrics given discrepancies between urine output and weight change.[79] Further studies are warranted in this field, especially focusing on novel and more reliable metrics of DR.

How to Improve Diuretic Response?

Currently there is no one-size-fits-all approach to the treatment of CRS (**Table 3**).

Diuretics are known to be associated with adverse outcomes and the DOSE trial failed to demonstrate adjunctive clinical benefits (beyond initial decongestion) with different dose or mode of administration.[26] Also, biomarker-guided therapy approaches have reported conflicting results.[80,81]

Torasemide is still underused in clinical practice, although it has a favorable pharmacologic profile (increased bioavailability and efficacy) compared with furosemide. Novel evidences suggested that torsemide may have antifibrotic properties, activating the enzymes involved in procollagen type I cleavage.[82,83] Observational data from the TOrasemide In Congestive Heart Failure (TORIC) study showed that chronic HF patients treated with torsemide had less frequently hypokalemia and improved survival.[84] However other studies suggested that torsemide-treated patients are generally sicker and have a worse outcome.[85,86] This seems to be largely related to confounding factors because, generally, torsemide is a second-line treatment, given to patients who do not respond to furosemide. In a recent subanalysis of the ASCEND-HF trial, up to 13% of subjects received torsemide. According to previous findings, torsemide-treated subjects had a higher risk profile with lower blood pressure and left ventricle ejection fraction and higher sCr and natriuretic peptides levels. Subjects in the torsemide group had nominally lower 30-day mortality or HF hospitalization, and 180-day mortality events in adjusted analysis.[87] Randomized prospective studies are still needed to ascertain the safety and the efficacy of this drug.

Combination therapy with thiazide-like diuretics such as metolazone is another option for patients with advanced HF and diuretic resistance.

Table 3
Therapeutic targets in cardiorenal syndrome

Target	Treatment	Pitfalls
Congestion	Diuretics	High doses associated with adverse outcomes
		No consensus about metric of DR
	Dopamine	No impact on clinical efficacy and outcomes
	Ultrafiltration	Not effective on renal function
		High treatment-related adverse events
	Peritoneal dialysis	Few data from clinical trials
		Experience limited to refractory HF
		High treatment-related adverse events
Neurohormonal activation	ACEI/ARBs	Contraindicated in patients with bilateral renal artery stenosis or sCr 2.5 mg/dL
		Need to reach target dose
	LCZ 696?	No data in real-world patients
Adenosine release	Rolofylline?	Clinical efficacy but unacceptable high rate of adverse events in clinical trials (seizures or stroke)
AVP release	Tolvaptan?	Clinical efficacy but no effect on outcomes
Anemia	Iron supplements?	No specific studies on CRS
Reduced cardiac output or renal hypoperfusion	Inotropes?	Increase of mortality and/or adverse events in clinical trials
Increased renal venous pressure	Vasodilators?	No data with nitrates
		Nesiritide does not worsen renal function but is associated with just a mild improvement of symptoms and no effect on outcomes
Inflammation and fibrosis	ACEI/ARBs	Contraindicated in patients with bilateral renal artery stenosis or sCr 2.5 mg/dL
		Need to reach target dose
	Immunomodulatory agents?	Still in early stage of development

Abbreviation: ACEI/ARBs, angiotensin-converting enzyme inhibitor/angiotensin receptor blockers; AVP, arginine vasopressine; LCZ696, neprilysin inhibitor sacubitril (AHU377) and the ARB valsartan.

Metolazone may enhance diuresis and natriuresis, although its use is balanced by potential adverse effects, such as deterioration of renal function and electrolyte disturbances, particularly hypokalemia.[88,89] No large placebo-controlled studies of metolazone have been performed, yet metolazone is used widely in clinical experience.

Tolvaptan is an oral selective vasopressin V2 antagonist aquaretic agent. In the Efficacy of Vasopressin Antagonism in Heart Failure Outcome Study With Tolvaptan (EVEREST) trial, this drug did not improve postdischarge outcome. However, it resulted in short-term benefits such as reduction of body weight and symptoms relief while preserving renal function.[90,91] Two ongoing clinical trials, Targeting Acute Congestion With Tolvaptan in Congestive Heart Failure (TACTICS) and Study to Evaluate Challenging Responses to Therapy in Congestive Heart Failure (SECRET of CHF), have been designed to confirm these findings.[92]

Recently, a novel approach with triple-therapy, including loop diuretics, oral vasopressin antagonists, and natriuretic doses of MRAs (MicroRNA), has been proposed. This drug regimen may lead to enhanced decongestion but the safety and efficacy needs to be evaluated in clinical trials.[93]

In addition, high-dose spironolactone may improve diuresis and congestion relief in AHF patients. This approach is currently undergoing investigation in the randomized, double-blind, placebo-controlled Aldosterone Targeted Neurohormonal Combined With Natriuresis Therapy-HF (ATHENA-HF) trial (NCT02235077). This study is evaluating the effect of high-dose MRA on N-terminal of the prohormone brain natriuretic petide (NT-proBNP) changes and several other measures of congestion relief.

Low-dose dopamine may induce renal vasodilation and increase urine output without worsening renal function. Despite data from small studies suggesting that dopamine enhances renal function,[94] low-dose dopamine added to standard diuretic treatment was not associated with any benefit in fluid loss and renal function in the Renal Optimization Strategies Evaluation in Acute Heart Failure (ROSE-AHF) trial.[95]

The impact of high dose of dobutamine or other inotropes in the treatment of renal dysfunction in still unclear.[96,97] Although preliminary data in subjects with advanced HF showed a decrease in sCr and an increase in creatinine clearance after infusion of levosimendan,[98] there is currently no evidence for a specific drug for the treatment and prevention of the CRS.

Venous-venous ultrafiltration (UF) has some advantages compared with loop diuretics because it allows continuous fluid removal with potentially less neurohormonal activation. Early studies demonstrated greater fluid loss and a reduction in HF rehospitalization rates in UF-treated patients compared with diuretic-based strategies.[99,100] However, the Cardiorenal Rescue Study in Acute Decompensated Heart Failure (CARRESS-HF) study reported worse outcomes with UF compared with pharmacological treatment, mainly due to an increase of sCr and an excess of treatment-related complications.[101] Also, the recent Aquapheresis vs Intravenous Diuretics and Hospitalization for Heart Failure (AVOID-HF) trial failed to demonstrate a clear benefit of UF compared with loop diuretics. Although the study showed a trend toward a longer time to first HF event and fewer cardiovascular events in the UF group, procedure-related complications were significantly higher in UF-treated patients. In addition, the trial was closed prematurely due to slow enrollment rate (27.5% of prespecified sample size) and, therefore, was largely unpowered to draw firm conclusions about clinical outcomes.[102] Further investigations on a larger population are needed and, currently, UF use is reserved for patients unresponsive to diuretics.

Peritoneal dialysis (PD) is an emerging potential treatment of palliative long-term care in patients with advanced HF and severe renal dysfunction. PD harnesses a physiological process of UF and sodium extraction through the peritoneal membrane. Being a home-based therapy, PD may offer potential advantages with respect to quality of life compared with routine community-based HD. However, patient compliance and family or caregiver support are mandatory before planning PD. PD-related complications such as infections, catheter malfunction, and hernias are relatively common and may have a strong impact on quality of life and outcomes in patients with advanced HF. Few clinical trials have investigated the role of PD in subjects with CRS. A recent study of 126 subjects with chronic refractory HF demonstrated a reduction of in-hospital days for AHF in PD-treated patients with acceptable adverse event rates (1 peritonitis episode in 26.2 patient months).[103] Smaller studies showed improvements in patients' clinical and functional status with PD compared with usual care.[104,105] Based on currently available data, PD may represent an option for patients with refractory HF and CRS.

Investigational Therapies

Ularitide is the synthetic analogue of urodilatin, a renal natriuretic peptide, which is involved in regulating renal hemodynamics, fluids, and sodium excretion. In the Safety and Efficacy of an Intravenous Placebo-Controlled Randomized Infusion of

Ularitide in a Prospective Double-Blind Study (SIRIUS) II trial, ularitide given at the dosage of 15 ng/Kg/min demonstrated a significant improvement of systemic hemodynamics and renal function metrics. A phase III study, the TRial of Ularitide's Efficacy and safety in patients with Acute Heart Failure (TRUE-AHF) is currently ongoing (NCT01661634).

Serelaxin is a vasodilator with antioxidative, antiinflammatory, and connective tissue–regulating properties. In the recent RELAXin in Acute Heart Failure (RELAX-AHF) trial, serelaxin treatment resulted in better dyspnea relief, improvement of clinical signs of congestion, and renal biomarkers profile. Notably, these clinical benefits have been translated in a significant reduction of 37% for 180-day mortality.[106] Possible explanations of this survival improvement may be at least partially attributed to the renal protective properties of serelaxin. Indeed, a subanalysis of the RELAX-AHF trial showed that serelaxin was associated with significantly lower sCr and CysC levels in the first 5 days after enrollment compared with placebo. Moreover, episodes of WRF were reduced in the serelaxin group, resulting in better 6-month outcomes.[107] Serelaxin demonstrated a direct impact on renal hemodynamics in a study of subjects with chronic HF. In serelaxin-treated subjects, renal plasma flow increased from baseline with 8 to 24 hours of infusion (change 29% serelaxin vs 14% placebo; P = .0386), without significant variations of GFR.[108] This renal vasodilating effect may unload the glomerulus by both renal afferent and efferent vasodilation. Although subjects with severe renal dysfunction were excluded from the abovementioned clinical trials, these observations may support the possible role of serelaxin in the treatment of CRS. A larger trial, the RELAX-AHF-II (NCT01870778), has been designed to confirm the survival benefit observed in previous studies and is currently in the recruiting phase. The entry criteria for this trial include an eGFR from 25 to 75 mL/min/1.73 m2.

The treatment and prevention of CRS remain targets of primary importance in HF clinical research. The preliminary promising results of serelaxin suggest that a treatment aimed at organ protection can improve prognosis and may have beneficial effects on CRS.

SUMMARY

In patients with advanced HF, renal dysfunction is an important comorbidity and has a major role in disease progression and may influence management options. Despite several limitations, sCr and GFR remain cornerstone diagnostic tests for the evaluation of renal function. Novel biomarkers may allow incremental discrimination of early AKI and may partially complement traditional markers if validated in subsequent robust analyses. Currently, there is no specific treatment of CRS in general; however, certain patients may benefit from different approaches, including addition of tolvaptan and/or triple therapy with loop diuretics, thiazides, and mineralocorticoid-receptor antagonists. However, novel therapeutics currently under investigation have shown favorable preliminary results in clinical trials and may be an future option to improve treatment responsiveness and outcomes.

REFERENCES

1. Mosterd A, Hoes AW. Clinical epidemiology of heart failure. Heart 2007;93:1137–46.
2. Aaronson KD, Schwartz JS, Chen TM, et al. Development and prospective validation of a clinical index to predict survival in ambulatory patients referred for cardiac transplant evaluation. Circulation 1997;95:2660–7.
3. Yancy CW, Jessup M, Bozkurt B, et al. 2013 ACCF/AHA guideline for the management of heart failure: a report of the American College of Cardiology Foundation/American Heart Association Task Force on Practice Guidelines. J Am Coll Cardiol 2013;62:e147–239.
4. McMurray JJ, Adamopoulos S, Anker SD, et al. ESC guidelines for the diagnosis and treatment of acute and chronic heart failure 2012: The Task Force for the Diagnosis and Treatment of Acute and Chronic Heart Failure 2012 of the European Society of Cardiology. Developed in collaboration with the Heart Failure Association (HFA) of the ESC. Eur J Heart Fail 2012;14:803–69.
5. Greene SJ, Fonarow GC, Vaduganathan M, et al. The vulnerable phase after hospitalization for heart failure. Nat Rev Cardiol 2015;12:220–9.
6. Gheorghiade M, Vaduganathan M, Fonarow GC, et al. Rehospitalization for heart failure: problems and perspectives. J Am Coll Cardiol 2013;61:391–403.
7. Mozaffarian D, Benjamin EJ, Go AS, et al. Heart disease and stroke statistics–2015 update: a report from the American Heart Association. Circulation 2015;131:e29–322.
8. Chong VH, Singh J, Parry H, et al. Management of noncardiac comorbidities in chronic heart failure. Cardiovasc Ther 2015;33:300–15.
9. Wong CY, Chaudhry SI, Desai MM, et al. Trends in comorbidity, disability, and polypharmacy in heart failure. Am J Med 2011;124:136–43.
10. Ezekowitz J, McAlister FA, Humphries KH, et al. The association among renal insufficiency, pharmacotherapy, and outcomes in 6,427 patients

with heart failure and coronary artery disease. J Am Coll Cardiol 2004;44:1587–92.

11. Hage FG, Venkataraman R, Zoghbi GJ, et al. The scope of coronary heart disease in patients with chronic kidney disease. J Am Coll Cardiol 2009; 53:2129–40.

12. Damman K, Valente MA, Voors AA, et al. Renal impairment, worsening renal function, and outcome in patients with heart failure: an updated meta-analysis. Eur Heart J 2014;35:455–69.

13. Fonarow GC, Adams KF Jr, Abraham WT, et al. Risk stratification for in-hospital mortality in acutely decompensated heart failure: classification and regression tree analysis. JAMA 2005;293:572–80.

14. Lazzarini V, Bettari L, Bugatti S, et al. Can we prevent or treat renal dysfunction in acute heart failure? Heart Fail Rev 2012;17:291–303.

15. Palazzuoli A, Lombardi C, Ruocco G, et al. Chronic kidney disease and worsening renal function in acute heart failure: different phenotypes with similar prognostic impact? Eur Heart J Acute Cardiovasc Care 2015. [Epub ahead of print].

16. van Veldhuisen DJ, Ruilope LM, Maisel AS, et al. Biomarkers of renal injury and function: diagnostic, prognostic and therapeutic implications in heart failure. Eur Heart J 2015. [Epub ahead of print].

17. Hillege HL, Nitsch D, Pfeffer MA, et al. Renal function as a predictor of outcome in a broad spectrum of patients with heart failure. Circulation 2006;113: 671–8.

18. Ahmed A, Rich MW, Sanders PW, et al. Chronic kidney disease associated mortality in diastolic versus systolic heart failure: a propensity matched study. Am J Cardiol 2007;99:393–8.

19. Cleland JGF, Carubelli V, Castiello T, et al. Renal dysfunction in acute and chronic heart failure: prevalence, incidence and prognosis. Heart Failure Rev 2012;17:133–49.

20. Carubelli V, Metra M, Lombardi C, et al. Renal dysfunction in acute heart failure: epidemiology, mechanisms and assessment. Heart Fail Rev 2012;17:271–82.

21. Mentz RJ, Lewis EF. Epidemiology of cardiorenal syndrome. Heart Fail Clin 2010;6:333–46.

22. Givertz MM, Postmus D, Hillege HL, et al. Renal function trajectories and clinical outcomes in acute heart failure. Circ Heart Fail 2014;7:59–67.

23. Smith GL, Lichtman JH, Bracken MB, et al. Renal impairment and outcomes in heart failure: systematic review and meta-analysis. J Am Coll Cardiol 2006;47:1987–96.

24. Damman K, Navis G, Voors AA, et al. Worsening renal function and prognosis in heart failure: systematic review and meta-analysis. J Card Fail 2007;13:599–608.

25. Metra M, Nodari S, Parrinello G, et al. Worsening renal function in patients hospitalised for acute heart failure: clinical implications and prognostic significance. Eur J Heart Fail 2008;10:188–95.

26. Felker GM, Lee KL, Bull DA, et al. Diuretic strategies in patients with acute decompensated heart failure. N Engl J Med 2011;364:797–805.

27. Metra M, Davison B, Bettari L, et al. Is worsening renal function an ominous prognostic sign in patients with acute heart failure? The role of congestion and its interaction with renal function. Circ Heart Fail 2012;5:54–62.

28. Ronco C, McCullough P, Anker SD, et al. Cardiorenal syndromes: report from the consensus conference of the acute dialysis quality initiative. Eur Heart J 2010;31:703–11.

29. Mentz RJ, O'Connor CM. Pathophysiology and clinical evaluation of acute heart failure. Nat Rev Cardiol 2016;13(1):28–35.

30. von Haehling S, Anker SD. Cardio-renal anemia syndrome. Contrib Nephrol 2011;171:266–73.

31. National Kidney Foundation. K/DOQI clinical practice guidelines for chronic kidney disease: evaluation, classification, and stratification. Am J Kidney Dis 2002;39:S1–266.

32. Levey AS, Stevens LA, Schmid CH, et al. A new equation to estimate glomerular filtration rate. Ann Intern Med 2009;150:604–12.

33. Levey AS, Bosch JP, Lewis JB, et al. A more accurate method to estimate glomerular filtration rate from serum creatinine: a new prediction equation. Modification of Diet in Renal Disease Study Group. Ann Intern Med 1999;130:461–70.

34. Stevens LA, Coresh J, Greene T, et al. Assessing kidney function–measured and estimated glomerular filtration rate. N Engl J Med 2006;354:2473–83.

35. Waikar SS, Bonventre JV. Creatinine kinetics and the definition of acute kidney injury. J Am Soc Nephrol 2009;20:672–9.

36. Bellomo R, Ronco C, Kellum JA, et al, Acute Dialysis Quality Initiative workgroup. Acute renal failure - definition, outcome measures, animal models, fluid therapy and information technology needs: the Second International Consensus Conference of the Acute Dialysis Quality Initiative (ADQI) Group. Crit Care 2004;8:R204–12.

37. Mehta RL, Kellum JA, Shah SV, et al, Acute Kidney Injury Network. Acute Kidney Injury Network: report of an initiative to improve outcomes in acute kidney injury. Crit Care 2007;11:R31.

38. Schrier RW. Blood urea nitrogen and serum creatinine: not married in heart failure. Circ Heart Fail 2008;1:2–5.

39. O'Connor CM, Mentz RJ, Cotter G, et al. The PROTECT in-hospital risk model: 7-day outcome in patients hospitalized with acute heart failure and renal dysfunction. Eur J Heart Fail 2012;14:605–12.

40. Lombardi C, Carubelli V, Rovetta R, et al. Prognostic value of serial measurements of blood urea

nitrogen in ambulatory patients with chronic heart failure. Panminerva Med 2016;58(1):8–15.

41. Grubb A. Diagnostic value of analysis of cystatin C and protein HC in biological fluids. Clin Nephrol 1992;38(Suppl 1):S20–7.

42. Inker LA, Schmid CH, Tighiouart H, et al. Estimating glomerular filtration rate from serum creatinine and cystatin C. N Engl J Med 2012; 367:20–9.

43. Lassus JP, Nieminen MS, Peuhkurinen K, et al. Markers of renal function and acute kidney injury in acute heart failure: definitions and impact on outcomes of the cardiorenal syndrome. Eur Heart J 2010;31:2791–8.

44. Damman K, van der Harst P, Smilde TD, et al. Use of cystatin C levels in estimating renal function and prognosis in patients with chronic systolic heart failure. Heart 2012;98:319–24.

45. Tang WH, Dupont M, Hernandez AF, et al. Comparative assessment of short-term adverse events in acute heart failure with cystatin C and other estimates of renal function: results from the ASCEND-HF trial. JACC Heart Fail 2015;3:40–9.

46. Haase M, Devarajan P, Haase-Fielitz A, et al. The outcome of neutrophil gelatinase-associated lipocalin-positive subclinical acute kidney injury: a multicenter pooled analysis of prospective studies. J Am Coll Cardiol 2011;57:1752–61.

47. Damman K, van Veldhuisen DJ, Navis G, et al. Urinary neutrophil gelatinase associated lipocalin (NGAL), a marker of tubular damage, is increased in patients with chronic heart failure. Eur J Heart Fail 2008;10:997–1000.

48. Palazzuoli A, Ruocco G, Pellegrini M, et al. Comparison of neutrophil gelatinase-associated lipocalin versus B-Type natriuretic peptide and cystatin c to predict early acute kidney injury and outcome in patients with acute heart failure. Am J Cardiol 2015; 116:104–11.

49. Ichimura T, Bonventre JV, Bailly V, et al. Kidney injury molecule-1 (KIM-1), a putative epithelial cell adhesion molecule containing a novel immunoglobulin domain, is up-regulated in renal cells after injury. J Biol Chem 1998;273:4135–42.

50. Liangos O, Perianayagam MC, Vaidya VS, et al. Urinary N-acetyl-beta-(D)-glucosaminidase activity and kidney injury molecule-1 level are associated with adverse outcomes in acute renal failure. J Am Soc Nephrol 2007;18:904–12.

51. van Timmeren MM, Bakker SJ, Vaidya VS, et al. Tubular kidney injury molecule-1 in protein-overload nephropathy. Am J Physiol Renal Physiol 2006;291:F456–64.

52. Damman K, Van Veldhuisen DJ, Navis G, et al. Tubular damage in chronic systolic heart failure is associated with reduced survival independent of glomerular filtration rate. Heart 2010;96:1297–302.

53. Damman K, Masson S, Hillege HL, et al. Tubular damage and worsening renal function in chronic heart failure. JACC Heart Fail 2013;1:417–24.

54. Grodin JL, Perez AL, Wu Y, et al. Circulating kidney injury molecule-1 levels in acute heart failure: insights from the ASCEND-HF trial (acute study of clinical effectiveness of nesiritide in decompensated heart failure). JACC Heart Fail 2015;3: 777–85.

55. Emmens JE, Ter Maaten JM, Matsue Y, et al. Plasma kidney injury molecule-1 in heart failure: renal mechanisms and clinical outcome. Eur J Heart Fail 2015. [Epub ahead of print].

56. Nauta FL, Boertien WE, Bakker SJ, et al. Glomerular and tubular damage markers are elevated in patients with diabetes. Diabetes Care 2011;34: 975–81.

57. Hamada Y, Kanda T, Anzai T, et al. N-acetyl-beta-D-glucosaminidase is not a predictor, but an indicator of kidney injury in patients with cardiac surgery. J Med 1999;30:329–36.

58. Damman K, Masson S, Hillege HL, et al. Clinical outcome of renal tubular damage in chronic heart failure. Eur Heart J 2011;32:2705–12.

59. Metra M, Cotter G, Gheorghiade M, et al. The role of the kidney in heart failure. Eur Heart J 2012;33: 2135–42.

60. Verbrugge FH, Dupont M, Shao Z, et al. Novel urinary biomarkers in detecting acute kidney injury, persistent renal impairment, and all-cause mortality following decongestive therapy in acute decompensated heart failure. J Card Fail 2013;19:621–8.

61. Veerkamp JH, Paulussen RJ, Peeters RA, et al. Detection, tissue distribution and (sub)cellular localization of fatty acid-binding protein types. Mol Cell Biochem 1990;98:11–8.

62. Katagiri D, Doi K, Honda K, et al. Combination of two urinary biomarkers predicts acute kidney injury after adult cardiac surgery. Ann Thorac Surg 2012; 93:577–83.

63. Ferguson MA, Vaidya VS, Waikar SS, et al. Urinary liver-type fatty acid-binding protein predicts adverse outcomes in acute kidney injury. Kidney Int 2010;77:708–14.

64. Shirakabe A, Hata N, Kobayashi N, et al. Serum heart-type fatty acid-binding protein level can be used to detect acute kidney injury on admission and predict an adverse outcome in patients with acute heart failure. Circ J 2015;79:119–28.

65. Ahmad T, Fiuzat M, Felker GM, et al. Novel biomarkers in chronic heart failure. Nat Rev Cardiol 2012;9:347–59.

66. Ahmad T, Fiuzat M, Pencina MJ, et al. Charting a roadmap for heart failure biomarker studies. JACC Heart Fail 2014;2(5):477–88.

67. Han WK, Wagener G, Zhu Y, et al. Urinary biomarkers in the early detection of acute kidney injury

after cardiac surgery. Clin J Am Soc Nephrol 2009; 4:873–82.

68. Coca SG, Garg AX, Thiessen-Philbrook H, et al. Urinary biomarkers of AKI and mortality 3 years after cardiac surgery. J Am Soc Nephrol 2014;25: 1063–71.

69. Ng LL, Sandhu JK, Narayan H, et al. Proenkephalin and prognosis after acute myocardial infarction. J Am Coll Cardiol 2014;63:280–9.

70. Felker GM, Mentz RJ. Diuretics and ultrafiltration in acute decompensated heart failure. J Am Coll Cardiol 2012;59:2145–53.

71. Metra M, Bugatti S, Bettari L, et al. Can we improve the treatment of congestion in heart failure? Expert Opin Pharmacother 2011;12:1369–79.

72. Ellison DH. Diuretic therapy and resistance in congestive heart failure. Cardiology 2001;96:132–43.

73. ter Maaten JM, Valente MA, Damman K, et al. Diuretic response in acute heart failure-pathophysiology, evaluation, and therapy. Nat Rev Cardiol 2015;12:184–92.

74. Testani JM, Chen J, McCauley BD, et al. Potential effects of aggressive decongestion during the treatment of decompensated heart failure on renal function and survival. Circulation 2010;122:265–72.

75. Testani JM, Brisco MA, Turner JM, et al. Loop diuretic efficiency: a metric of diuretic responsiveness with prognostic importance in acute decompensated heart failure. Circ Heart Fail 2014;7: 261–70.

76. Valente MA, Voors AA, Damman K, et al. Diuretic response in acute heart failure: clinical characteristics and prognostic significance. Eur Heart J 2014; 35(19):1284–93.

77. ter Maaten JM, Dunning AM, Valente MA, et al. Diuretic response in acute heart failure-an analysis from ASCEND-HF. Am Heart J 2015;170:313–21.

78. Voors AA, Davison BA, Teerlink JR, et al. Diuretic response in patients with acute decompensated heart failure: characteristics and clinical outcome-an analysis from RELAX-AHF. Eur J Heart Fail 2014;16:1230–40.

79. Testani JM, Brisco MA, Kociol RD, et al. Substantial discrepancy between fluid and weight loss during acute decompensated heart failure treatment. Am J Med 2015;128:776–83.e4.

80. Shah MR, Califf RM, Nohria A, et al. The STARBRITE trial: a randomized, pilot study of B-type natriuretic peptide-guided therapy in patients with advanced heart failure. J Card Fail 2011;17:613–21.

81. Troughton RW, Frampton CM, Brunner-La Rocca HP, et al. Effect of B-type natriuretic peptide-guided treatment of chronic heart failure on total mortality and hospitalization: an individual patient meta-analysis. Eur Heart J 2014;35:1559–67.

82. Lopez B, Gonzalez A, Beaumont J, et al. Identification of a potential cardiac antifibrotic mechanism of torasemide in patients with chronic heart failure. J Am Coll Cardiol 2007;50:859–67.

83. Buggey J, Mentz RJ, Pitt B, et al. A reappraisal of loop diuretic choice in heart failure patients. Am Heart J 2015;169:323–33.

84. Cosin J, Diez J, TORIC investigators. Torasemide in chronic heart failure: results of the TORIC study. Eur J Heart Fail 2002;4:507–13.

85. Mentz RJ, Buggey J, Fiuzat M, et al. Torsemide versus furosemide in heart failure patients: insights from Duke University Hospital. J Cardiovasc Pharmacol 2015;65:438–43.

86. Mentz RJ, Velazquez EJ, Metra M, et al. Comparative effectiveness of torsemide versus furosemide in heart failure patients: insights from the PROTECT trial. Future Cardiol 2015;11:585–95.

87. Mentz RJ, Hasselblad V, DeVore AD, et al. Torsemide versus furosemide in patients with acute heart failure (from the ASCEND-HF trial). Am J Cardiol 2016;117:404–11.

88. Rosenberg J, Gustafsson F, Galatius S, et al. Combination therapy with metolazone and loop diuretics in outpatients with refractory heart failure: an observational study and review of the literature. Cardiovasc Drugs Ther 2005;19:301–6.

89. Channer KS, McLean KA, Lawson-Matthew P, et al. Combination diuretic treatment in severe heart failure: a randomised controlled trial. Br Heart J 1994; 71:146–50.

90. Konstam MA, Gheorghiade M, Burnett JC, et al. Effects of oral tolvaptan in patients hospitalized for worsening heart failure: the EVEREST outcome trial. JAMA 2007;297:1319–31.

91. Gheorghiade M, Konstam MA, Burnett JC, et al. Short-term clinical effects of tolvaptan, an oral vasopressin antagonist, in patients hospitalized for heart failure: the EVEREST clinical status trials. JAMA 2007;297:1332–43.

92. Felker GM, Mentz RJ, Adams KF, et al. Tolvaptan in patients hospitalized with acute heart failure: rationale and design of the TACTICS and the SECRET of CHF trials. Circ Heart Fail 2015;8:997–1005.

93. Vaduganathan M, Mentz RJ, Greene SJ, et al. Combination decongestion therapy in hospitalized heart failure: loop diuretics, mineralocorticoid receptor antagonists and vasopressin antagonists. Expert Rev Cardiovasc Ther 2015;13:799–809.

94. Giamouzis G, Butler J, Starling RC, et al. Impact of dopamine infusion on renal function in hospitalized heart failure patients: results of the dopamine in acute decompensated heart failure (DAD-HF) trial. J Card Fail 2010;16:922–30.

95. Chen HH, Anstrom KJ, Givertz MM, et al. Low-dose dopamine or low-dose nesiritide in acute heart failure with renal dysfunction: the ROSE acute heart failure randomized trial. JAMA 2013;310: 2533–43.

96. Metra M, Bettari L, Carubelli V, et al. Use of inotropic agents in patients with advanced heart failure: lessons from recent trials and hopes for new agents. Drugs 2011;71:515–25.

97. Metra M, Bettari L, Carubelli V, et al. Old and new intravenous inotropic agents in the treatment of advanced heart failure. Prog Cardiovasc Dis 2011;54:97–106.

98. Zemljic G, Bunc M, Yazdanbakhsh AP, et al. Levosimendan improves renal function in patients with advanced chronic heart failure awaiting cardiac transplantation. J Card Fail 2007;13:417–21.

99. Bart BA, Boyle A, Bank AJ, et al. Ultrafiltration versus usual care for hospitalized patients with heart failure: the relief for acutely fluid-overloaded patients with decompensated congestive heart failure (RAPID-CHF) trial. J Am Coll Cardiol 2005;46: 2043–6.

100. Costanzo MR, Guglin ME, Saltzberg MT, et al. Ultrafiltration versus intravenous diuretics for patients hospitalized for acute decompensated heart failure. J Am Coll Cardiol 2007;49:675–83.

101. Bart BA, Goldsmith SR, Lee KL, et al. Ultrafiltration in decompensated heart failure with cardiorenal syndrome. N Engl J Med 2012;367:2296–304.

102. Costanzo MR, Negoianu D, Jaski BE, et al. Aquapheresis versus intravenous diuretics and hospitalizations for heart failure. JACC Heart Fail 2016;4(2):95–105.

103. Courivaud C, Kazory A, Crepin T, et al. Peritoneal dialysis reduces the number of hospitalization days in heart failure patients refractory to diuretics. Perit Dial Int 2014;34:100–8.

104. Koch M, Haastert B, Kohnle M, et al. Peritoneal dialysis relieves clinical symptoms and is well tolerated in patients with refractory heart failure and chronic kidney disease. Eur J Heart Fail 2012;14: 530–9.

105. Nunez J, Gonzalez M, Minana G, et al. Continuous ambulatory peritoneal dialysis as a therapeutic alternative in patients with advanced congestive heart failure. Eur J Heart Fail 2012;14:540–8.

106. Teerlink JR, Cotter G, Davison BA, et al. Serelaxin, recombinant human relaxin-2, for treatment of acute heart failure (RELAX-AHF): a randomised, placebo-controlled trial. Lancet 2013;381:29–39.

107. Metra M, Cotter G, Davison BA, et al. Effect of serelaxin on cardiac, renal, and hepatic biomarkers in the relaxin in acute heart failure (RELAX-AHF) development program: correlation with outcomes. J Am Coll Cardiol 2013;61:196–206.

108. Voors AA, Dahlke M, Meyer S, et al. Renal hemodynamic effects of serelaxin in patients with chronic heart failure: a randomized, placebo-controlled study. Circ Heart Fail 2014;7:994–1002.

Cardiohepatic Interactions
Implications for Management in Advanced Heart Failure

Akshay Pendyal, MD, Jill M. Gelow, MD, MPH*

KEYWORDS

- Chronic heart failure • Advanced heart failure • Hepatic fibrosis • Cirrhosis • Hepatitis C
- Liver disease • Heart transplantation • Mechanical circulatory support

KEY POINTS

- Liver disease is common in patients with advanced heart failure and can significantly impact morbidity and mortality.
- It is difficult to diagnose severe liver disease, including hepatic fibrosis and cirrhosis, in advanced heart failure based on history, physical examination, and imaging studies.
- Liver biopsy is the gold standard for diagnosis of hepatic fibrosis and cirrhosis in advanced heart failure.
- Liver disease has important implications for advanced heart failure therapies and should be considered in selecting patients for mechanical circulatory support and heart transplant.
- Hepatitis C is common, and strategies for treatment of hepatitis C in patients with advanced heart failure continue to evolve with the recent development of direct-acting antiviral agents.

Liver disease is a common sequela of advanced heart failure (HF; American College of Cardiology/American Heart Association stage D), ranging from mild reversible liver injury to hepatic fibrosis and, in its most severe form, cardiac cirrhosis.[1] Although it can be challenging to identify in patients with HF, the presence of liver disease has important implications for prognosis, medication management, mechanical circulatory support (MCS), and heart transplantation (HT).

In this review, a framework is provided for approaching liver disease in the advanced HF population. After a brief review of hepatic anatomy and the pathophysiology of liver disease in HF, the authors summarize the current understanding of chronic liver disease in HF and examine the implications of chronic liver disease for MCS and HT. Given the increasing prevalence of hepatitis C virus (HCV) and the recent development and approval of a new class of HCV therapeutics, specific considerations are included for the management of HCV in the advanced HF population.

HEPATIC ANATOMY AND PATHOPHYSIOLOGY

The liver receives 25% to 30% of the total cardiac output from 2 vascular sources, the hepatic artery and the portal vein. The portal vein carries nutrient-rich blood from the mesenteric and splenic veins and provides 70% of the hepatic blood flow. The hepatic artery, a branch of the celiac trunk, supplies oxygenated blood from the heart and lungs

Disclosure Statement: The authors have nothing to disclose.
Knight Cardiovascular Institute, Oregon Health and Science University, 3181 Southwest Sam Jackson Park Road, UHN 62, Portland, OR 97239, USA
* Corresponding author.
E-mail address: gelowj@ohsu.edu

Heart Failure Clin 12 (2016) 349–361
http://dx.doi.org/10.1016/j.hfc.2016.03.011
1551-7136/16/$ – see front matter
© 2016 Elsevier Inc. All rights reserved.

and accounts for the remainder of hepatic blood flow.[2] On entering the liver, blood from the portal vein and hepatic artery drains into the endothelium-lined hepatic sinusoids. Plasma is filtered through the sinusoidal endothelium to perfuse the hepatocytes, which are rich with metabolic activity. Blood then returns to the inferior vena cava (IVC) through the hepatic veins.[2]

There are 2 models used to describe the functional unit of the liver: the classic lobule (**Fig. 1**A) and the liver acinus (**Fig. 1**B).[2] The classic lobule is a hexagonal structure organized around a central venule, a branch of the hepatic vein. The portal tracts, comprising the hepatic artery, portal vein, bile ducts, lymphatics, and nerves, are located at the corners of the hexagon. In contrast, the liver acinus describes the liver parenchyma in zones. Hepatocytes in zone 1 are closest to the portal triad; thus, they receive the richest supply of oxygen and nutrients but are also more likely to be damaged by drugs and toxins because they are exposed to the highest concentrations. The hepatocytes in zone 3 are near the central vein and have a relatively poor supply of oxygen. These hepatocytes are more susceptible to damage from hypoxia and venous congestion.[2]

Liver chemistries, or liver function tests (LFTs), provide important information for diagnosis and monitoring. Alanine aminotransferase (ALT) and aspartate aminotransferase (AST) are present in hepatocytes, and elevation of these transaminases signifies hepatocellular injury or necrosis. Elevations in alkaline phosphatase (AP), γ-glutamyl transferase, and bilirubin are reflective of obstructive or cholestatic disease. Low albumin and prolonged prothrombin time (PT) indicate impaired hepatic synthetic function.[2]

The liver's dual blood supply provides substantial physiologic reserve. When portal blood flow is reduced, the liver compensates by vasodilating hepatic arterioles to maintain blood flow, a response that is mediated by adenosine released from injured hepatocytes.[3] The liver is able to increase oxygen extraction to allow up to 95% of oxygen to be extracted in a single pass.[4] Given this reserve, hypotension alone is typically not enough to precipitate ischemic hepatitis.[3]

Ischemic hepatitis is characterized biochemically by a rapid increase in AST and ALT up to 10 to 20 times the upper limit of normal within 24 hours of a hemodynamic insult, and histopathologically by severe hepatocellular injury causing centrilobular (zone 3) necrosis. Although more commonly associated with acute cardiogenic shock, ischemic hepatitis can develop in patients with chronic HF.[4,5] The degree and duration of hemodynamic derangement needed to precipitate acute ischemic hepatitis in HF differ depending on the chronicity of HF and the extent of compensation.[6] For example, in a patient with chronic HF who has been exposed to chronic passive congestion of the liver, a small decrease in blood pressure or cardiac output may be enough to result in ischemic hepatitis. In contrast, in patients with cardiogenic shock due to acute HF or compensated chronic HF without chronic passive congestion, a more profound degree of hypoperfusion is required to cause ischemic hepatitis.[3,6]

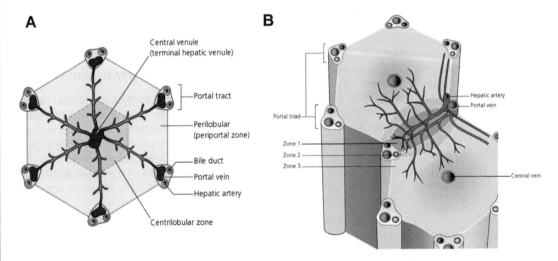

Fig. 1. The functional unit of the liver. (*A*) The classic lobule where the portal tracts form the corners of a hexagon centered around the central vein. (*B*) The liver acinus where hepatocytes in zone 1 are closest to the portal triad and hepatocytes on zone 3 are closest to the central vein. (*From* Nash K. Hepatology: clinical cases uncovered. Hoboken (NJ): Wiley-Blackwell; 2011; with permission.)

Ischemic hepatitis does not necessarily result in chronic liver disease. In HF, chronic liver disease develops as a result of chronically elevated right-sided filling pressures, which lead to increased hepatic venous pressure and passive hepatic congestion. Decreased hepatic blood flow and hypoxia also play a clear role in the development of chronic liver disease in HF.[7] Oxidative stress, upregulated pro-inflammatory cytokines, and thrombosis contribute, although the exact mechanisms are not clear.[8–10]

LIVER DISEASE IN ADVANCED HEART FAILURE

Patients with HF may develop transient mild liver injury, often termed congestive hepatopathy, due to passive congestion and manifested by elevated LFTs or even hepatomegaly and ascites. With optimization of HF, LFT abnormalities improve. Identifying the point at which benign reversible liver injury due to congestive hepatopathy transforms into chronic fibrosis and, ultimately, cirrhosis in HF patients is challenging but important. Mild liver injury and reversible fibrosis in advanced HF patients may improve with MCS and HT, whereas patients with severe fibrosis and cirrhosis are at high risk for morbidity and mortality, precluding these therapies.[11]

Diagnosis of Chronic Liver Disease in Heart Failure

History, physical examination, laboratory assessment, and imaging are helpful in diagnosing chronic liver disease in advanced HF, but each possesses its own challenges. The symptoms and physical examination findings of chronic liver disease and HF overlap. Although elevated LFTs are common in advanced HF, they are not specific for fibrosis; conversely, normal LFTs can be seen in the presence of severe fibrosis or cirrhosis.[12,13] The reported prevalence of abnormal liver chemistries in patients hospitalized with HF is variable (**Table 1**).[14–18] A cholestatic or obstructive pattern has most commonly been described in HF and is associated with moderate to severe tricuspid regurgitation (TR), elevated central venous pressure, and objective evidence of right-sided volume overload with elevated jugular venous pressure and peripheral edema.[19,20] Imaging with ultrasound or computed tomography (CT) can be helpful in diagnosing chronic liver disease in patients with HF.[21] However, when compared with liver

Table 1
Prevalence of abnormal liver function tests in patients hospitalized for acute heart failure: post-hoc analyses of randomized controlled trials

Source Study	Prevalence of LFT Abnormalities (%)		Additional Findings
EVEREST[14] Tolvaptan vs placebo (n = 2061)	Albumin AP Bilirubin ALT AST	17 23 26 21 21	Persistent LFT abnormalities were common at hospital discharge Lower albumin and higher total bilirubin at baseline were associated with increased mortality
SURVIVE[15] Levosimendan vs dobutamine (n = 1134)	AP ALT AST	21 25 33	Abnormal AP was associated with congestion Abnormal AST and ALT were associated with clinical hypoperfusion and increased mortality
ESCAPE[16] Clinical vs pulmonary artery catheter-guided therapy (n = 346)	Albumin Bilirubin ALT AST	24 36 24 24	Elevated total bilirubin was associated with lower cardiac index and higher central venous pressure Elevated MELD-XI was associated with worse outcomes
Pre-RELAX-AHF[17] Relaxin vs placebo (n = 234)	Albumin AP Bilirubin ALT AST	25 12 19 12 21	AST and ALT were associated with worse outcomes
ASCEND-HF[18] Nesiritide vs placebo (n = 4228)	Bilirubin ALT AST	42 22 30	Elevated bilirubin was associated with worse outcomes

biopsy, CT or ultrasound had a low sensitivity (30%) and poor negative predictive value (21%) for the diagnosis of hepatic fibrosis in an advanced HF population.[12]

Given these diagnostic challenges, liver biopsy remains the gold standard for diagnosing chronic liver disease in advanced HF patients.[21] Liver biopsy is most often performed via the transjugular approach in patients with HF; this approach is generally safe and can be performed simultaneously with right heart catheterization.[21,22] Sampling error and variation in interpretation must be considered when reviewing biopsy results. In selected cases, percutaneous or open biopsy may be required. Transjugular liver biopsy also allows for the measurement of hepatic hemodynamics. Hepatic venous pressure gradient (HVPG) estimates the pressure gradient between the portal vein and the IVC and helps to diagnosis and quantify portal hypertension. A normal HVPG is 1 to 5 mm Hg. Portal hypertension is suggested if the HVPG is 6 mm Hg or greater.[23]

Hepatic fibrosis and cirrhosis: histopathology, prevalence, and clinical characteristics

The histopathologic hallmarks of liver disease due to HF are chronic passive congestion (central vein and sinusoidal dilation, termed "nutmeg liver" in its most severe form) and centrilobular (zone 3) necrosis.[5] Over time, passive congestion and centrilobular necrosis progress to hepatic fibrosis and, ultimately, cardiac cirrhosis.[5] A retrospective study of advanced HF patients referred for liver biopsy found that most patients had congestion, centrilobular fibrosis and necrosis, and sinusoidal dilation (**Fig. 2**A).[12] Hepatic fibrosis of any severity was identified in 80% of patients, with bridging fibrosis (**Fig. 2**B) or cirrhosis occurring in 37% of patients.[12] In this study, patients with biopsy-proven fibrosis were more likely to have a mixed or obstructive pattern of LFT abnormalities, moderate to severe TR, and decreased renal function.[12] There was no association between hepatic fibrosis and gender, age, cause of cardiomyopathy, duration of symptoms, right or left ventricular dysfunction, cardiac filling pressures, HCV status, or abnormal abdominal imaging.[12] In another series of patients with cardiac hepatopathy, no correlation was found between hepatic fibrosis and cardiac or hepatic hemodynamics.[13]

The current understanding of the prevalence and risk factors for hepatic fibrosis in HF is limited, in part due to the heterogeneous nature of HF pathophysiology and the selection bias of patients referred for liver biopsy. In addition, interpretation of biopsy specimens in both clinical practice and research is inconsistent, with most pathologists using scoring criteria that were developed for noncardiac liver disease. Standardizing interpretation of hepatic biopsies in HF patients is important as we strive to advance the understanding of liver disease in this population. Dai and colleagues[24] recently proposed a congestive hepatic fibrosis scoring system for liver disease resulting from HF (**Fig. 3**).

In general, suspicion for chronic liver disease should be heightened in patients with advanced HF, particularly in those with right HF, restrictive cardiomyopathies, congenital heart disease, abnormal LFTs or liver imaging, heavy alcohol use, or HCV.[11] Given the challenges in diagnosis and the lack of correlation of biopsy-proven fibrosis with clinical characteristics, it may be prudent to have a low threshold for transjugular liver biopsy, particularly for patients undergoing evaluation for advanced therapies.

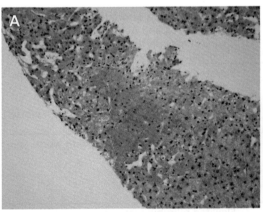 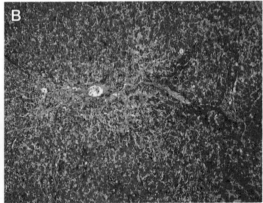

Fig. 2. (*A*) Liver biopsy with pericentral congestion, hepatocyte necrosis, and sinusoidal dilatation (hematoxylin-eosin, original magnification ×). (*B*) Liver biopsy with bridging fibrosis (trichrome, original magnification ×). (*Courtesy of* Jonathan Glickman, MD, MPH, Boston, MA.)

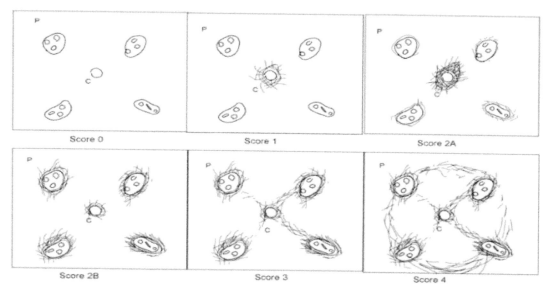

Fig. 3. Congestive fibrosis scoring system: score 0, no fibrosis; score 1, central zone fibrosis only; score 2A, central zone and portal fibrosis, with accentuation of fibrosis in the central zone; score 2B, moderate portal fibrosis and central zone fibrosis, with accentuation of fibrosis in the portal zone; score 3, bridging fibrosis; and score 4, cirrhosis. C, central venule; P, portal triad. (*From* Dai DF, Swanson PE, Krieger EV, et al. Congestive hepatic fibrosis score: a novel histologic assessment of clinical severity. Mod Pathol 2014;27(12):1554; with permission.)

Prognosis of Liver Disease in Heart Failure

Multiple studies have shown an association between elevated LFTs and poor prognosis in HF, but the results have been variable with respect to the specific LFTs identified and associated outcomes.[14–18] Clinical risk scores, such as the Model for End Stage Liver Disease (MELD) and the Model for End Stage Liver Disease Excluding INR (international normalized ratio; MELD-XI), are also helpful for prognostication in HF.[25,26] MELD uses serum bilirubin, creatinine, and the INR or PT to predict survival. Given that many patients with HF are treated with systemic anticoagulation (thus limiting the utility of INR), MELD-XI is a modified risk score that includes only serum bilirubin and serum creatinine. In advanced HF patients undergoing evaluation for HT, MELD score greater than 12 was associated with increased mortality at 1 year.[25] In patients hospitalized with HF, MELD-XI score 10 or greater was an independent predictor of cardiac death and all-cause mortality.[26] In the Evaluation Study of Congestive Heart Failure and Pulmonary Artery Catheter Effectiveness (ESCAPE) study, the 6-month event-free survival was 23.5% for patients in the high MELD-XI score group (≥16.8) compared with 46.2% for patients in the low MELD-XI score group.[16]

High-Risk Medications in Heart Failure and Liver Dysfunction

Hepatic dysfunction, whether primary or resulting from cardiac disease, can significantly alter the pharmacokinetics of many HF medications. Unfortunately, in hepatic dysfunction, serum drug levels and target effects are often unpredictable and do not correlate well with the specific cause of liver disease, its severity, or levels of LFTs. There are thus no readily generalizable rules for modifying drug dosing in patients with liver disease. Some medications used in advanced HF, such as lisinopril, spironolactone, milrinone, and dobutamine, require no specific dosage adjustments in liver dysfunction. Many other medications, however, do carry certain considerations in hepatic disease and are outlined in **Table 2**.

Hepatitis C and Its Role in Heart Failure

HCV represents a unique entity at the nexus of HF and liver disease. HCV is responsible for more than 4 million cases of chronic hepatitis in the United States and 170 million cases worldwide, and, if untreated, can result in cirrhosis.[27,28] New cases continue to arise, mainly due to transmission via intravenous drug use and sexual intercourse.[29] Genotypes 1a and 1b are the most prevalent HCV subtypes in the Western world, followed by genotypes 2 and 3.

Given the high prevalence of both HCV and HF, the 2 entities often coexist, although the true frequency of this is not known. In addition, it is unknown whether HCV accelerates the development of chronic liver disease in HF or vice versa. Interestingly, HCV has been implicated in the pathogenesis

Table 2
Commonly prescribed medications in advanced heart failure and their specific considerations with concomitant liver disease

Drug	Metabolism	Dose Adjustment in Liver Disease	Monitoring
Amiodarone	Undergoes hepatic metabolism via CYP2C8 and CYP3A4 to its active metabolite N-desethylamiodarone; also inhibits CYP2A6, CYP2C9, and CYP2D6	Modification is probably necessary with significant hepatic impairment. If transaminases exceed 3 times normal, decreasing the dose or even discontinuing the drug may be reasonable	Liver function tests should be obtained semiannually in patients with normal liver function, and likely more frequently in those with liver dysfunction
Warfarin	Undergoes hepatic metabolism, primarily via CYP2C9; minor pathways include CYP2C8, 2C18, 2C19, 1A2, and 3A4	In patients with hepatic impairment, the response to warfarin is enhanced by impaired native synthesis of clotting factors and decreased liver metabolism	Frequent INR monitoring is necessary
Losartan	Substrate of CYP2C9 and CYP3A4; weak inhibitor of CYP1A2 and CYP2C19; moderate inhibitor of CYP2C8 and CYP2C9. Extensive first-pass metabolism; oral bioavailability is 33%. Metabolized to active form via hepatic carboxylation	In patients with hepatic impairment, bioavailability is doubled and total clearances is halved; therefore, lower starting doses are recommended	As with angiotensin converting enzyme inhibitors, serum drug levels are not routinely obtained, but monitoring of renal function and electrolytes is recommended
Sodium nitroprusside	Nitroprusside is metabolized via combination with hemoglobin to form cyanmethemoglobin and cyanide ions. Cyanide is, in turn, converted via reaction with thiosulfate by the enzyme rhodanese, which is widely distributed in hepatic cells. Nitroprusside is completely excreted via the kidneys as thiocyanate	Due to the risk of cyanide toxicity, it should be used with extreme caution, as the mitochondrial enzyme rhodanese, which is present in abundance in the liver, can be dysfunctional or absent in hepatic impairment	Monitoring for cyanide toxicity via acid-base balance and mixed venous oxygen saturation is recommended
Statins	All statins undergo extensive hepatic metabolism, with CYP3A4 being the major enzyme responsible	Recent data suggest that statins are generally well tolerated in patients with chronic stable liver disease; in decompensated cirrhosis and acute liver failure, however, statins are contraindicated	Frequent monitoring of hepatic function, including liver enzymes and coagulation, is recommended
Torsemide	Undergoes mostly hepatic metabolism (~80%) via the cytochrome P450 system; volume of distribution (V_d) is approximately doubled in cirrhosis, and half-life elimination is doubled from ~3.5 h to 7–8 h	Prescribers should exercise caution to avoid fluid and electrolyte shifts, which may lead to hepatic encephalopathy	Frequent monitoring of renal function, blood pressure, and volume status is necessary

of coronary artery disease and nonischemic dilated cardiomyopathy.[30–32] One study examining more than 1300 patients with idiopathic chronic HF found circulating anti-HCV antibodies among HF patients at a significantly higher rate than that observed in the general population; moreover, HCV infection was more often associated with elevated serum markers of myocardial injury.[33] It is possible that chronic HCV infection predisposes individuals to the development of subclinical myocarditis, which in turn leads to the eventual development of dilated cardiomyopathy.

HCV infection also carries specific implications for treatment in the advanced HF population. Until relatively recently, treatment of chronic HCV infection most often centered on ribavirin and interferon (IFN)-based regimens, which are associated with prohibitive adverse cardiac effects.[34] The development and approval of multiple direct-acting antivirals (DAAs), however, have ushered in a new era in the treatment of HCV infection. These medications target specific steps within the HCV life cycle, disrupting viral replication and infection. DAAs can be categorized into nonstructural proteins 3/4A (NS3/4A) protease inhibitors, such as telaprevir, boceprevir, simeprevir, and paritaprevir; NS5B nucleoside polymerase inhibitors, such as sofosbuvir; NS5B nonnucleoside polymerase inhibitors, such as dasabuvir; and NS5A inhibitors, such as ledipasvir, ombitasvir, and daclatasvir. Some of these are offered in single- or fixed-dose combinations. Several treatment algorithms for chronic HCV infection exist for each genotype, ranging in duration from 8 to 24 weeks. On the whole, these new agents have proven remarkably effective, achieving sustained virologic response rates in excess of 80% in treatment-naïve patients—a response that is effectively tantamount to virologic cure.[35,36]

Potential adverse cardiac effects of these agents include bradyarrhythmias, especially when used in conjunction with amiodarone.[37] Reported cardiac drug-drug interactions include furosemide and warfarin.[38] Nevertheless, despite these concerns, given the improved safety profile and ease of administration of DAAs compared with IFN, serologic testing should be considered early in the evaluation of patients with advanced HF to facilitate timely treatment and minimize liver injury.

CHRONIC LIVER DISEASE AND ADVANCED HEART FAILURE THERAPIES
Chronic Liver Disease and Mechanical Circulatory Support

Preimplantation liver dysfunction is an important determinant of mortality risk following left ventricular assist device (LVAD) implantation and is associated with postoperative right HF and right ventricular assist device (RVAD) implantation.[39–41] Significant ascites on abdominal imaging and abnormal LFTs, particularly high preoperative bilirubin, have been associated with decreased survival after LVAD.[42,43] Preimplantation MELD and MELD-XI scores also impact post-LVAD outcomes. Increasing, MELD scores are associated with higher postoperative transfusion requirements.[39] Worse survival has been demonstrated for patients with MELD and MELD XI scores greater than or equal to 17.[39,40] In the INTERMACS (Interagency Registry for Mechanically Assisted Circulatory Support) cohort, the 6-month survival for patients with MELD scores greater than or equal to 17 was 67% ± 5% compared with 82% ± 3% in patients with MELD scores less than 17.[39] Some groups have published favorable experiences with LVAD implantation in patients with advanced hepatic disease; however, morbidity in these populations is high and includes vasoplegia, infection, gastrointestinal bleeding, need for dialysis, and right HF requiring RVAD.[44]

Given heterogeneity in patients referred for liver biopsy before LVAD and the fact that patients with significant hepatic fibrosis and cirrhosis are often declined LVAD implantation, data regarding outcomes after LVAD in patients with hepatic fibrosis on liver biopsy are limited.[12] A study of 16 patients undergoing liver biopsy because of concern for significant liver disease found 14 patients to have evidence of hepatic fibrosis but not cirrhosis. There were no differences in intensive care unit length of stay, hospital length of stay, and 1-year survival between these 14 patients and more than 200 patients who did not undergo liver biopsy, but there was an increase in gastrointestinal bleeding at 1 year.[45] Farr and colleagues[46] combined liver biopsy results with MELD-XI scores to create a liver risk score for 68 patients with suspected advanced liver disease undergoing HT and LVAD evaluation. The liver risk score was calculated as (fibrosis-on-biopsy + 1) × MELD-XI, where degree of fibrosis was scored on a scale of 0 to 4. Of the 68 patients, 52 patients were listed for HT, 8 underwent LVAD, 5 underwent biventricular assist device, and 1 underwent total artificial heart. A cutoff score of 45 was selected as an indicator of high risk. One-year survival after VAD surgery was 85.7% in low-risk patients with a liver risk score less than 45 compared with 57.1% in high-risk patients with a liver risk score greater than or equal to 45. Thus, in selected lower risk patients with some degree of hepatic fibrosis on liver biopsy, LVAD may be appropriate.

Chronic Liver Disease and Heart Transplantation

Advanced HF patients with cirrhosis have poor outcomes following HT.[47,48] Thus, cirrhosis is an absolute contraindication to isolated HT at most centers. The impact of lesser stages of liver disease on outcomes after HT is less clear. MELD and MELD-XI score are associated with worse outcomes after HT. In a single-center retrospective analysis of 617 patients undergoing HT, 1-year and 5-year survival, respectively, were 91.4% and 83.2% in patients with MELD scores less than 14 compared with 85.5% and 70.1% in patients with MELD scores greater than 20.[49] In an analysis of the United Network for Organ Sharing database, 30-day post-HT mortality increased from 3.7% in those with MELD-XI scores less than 5 to 28.0% in those with MELD-XI scores greater than 30.[50] MELD-XI score was also associated with posttransplant complications, including infections, stroke, dialysis, rejection, and prolonged hospitalization.[50]

Similar to the MCS literature, little is known regarding the association of specific liver biopsy findings with HT outcomes. Twenty-one patients who had liver biopsies available for review and who underwent HT at a single center over a 16-year period were studied. Increased fibrosis was identified in 19 of the 21 biopsies, including 13 with bridging fibrosis and 6 with regenerative nodules. Of the 21 patients, only 15 patients (71.4%) were alive at 1 year. Perioperative morbidity was high and included bleeding, infection, and liver failure.[51] In the study by Farr and colleagues,[46] 1-year survival after HT listing was 86.7% in risk low-risk patients with liver risk score less than 45, but 45.5% in high-risk patients with a liver risk score greater than or equal to 45. In selected low-risk patients with hepatic fibrosis on biopsy, HT may be reasonable.

For patients with cirrhosis or significant hepatic fibrosis, combined heart-liver transplantation may be possible. Reported outcomes for combined heart-liver transplantation have been favorable, and there may be a lower incidence of rejection because liver allografts are thought to enhance tolerance to other donor-specific allografts.[52,53] Heart-liver transplantation is particularly appealing for disorders such as familial transthyretin amyloidosis, where transplanting both organs could both ameliorate the cardiac abnormality and cure the underlying disorder.[54] The role of heart-liver transplantation in advanced HF patients with cirrhosis and treated HCV is unknown.

Hepatitis C and Advanced Heart Failure Therapies

Successful treatment of HCV infection following LVAD implantation has been reported, and HCV treatment may allow destination-therapy LVAD patients to become candidates for HT.[55] Patients with liver disease due to HCV may be thrombocytopenic with increased propensity for bleeding. LVADs may augment this risk due to the development of acquired von Willebrand disease and the need for therapeutic anticoagulation.[55,56] LVAD implantation itself may have an immunomodulatory effect that engenders higher levels of circulating HCV antibodies, and although the exact mechanism underlying this phenomenon remains unclear, it does underscore the importance of confirmatory nucleic acid testing (NAT) (ie, RNA polymerase chain reaction) in patients with advanced HF and positive HCV antibody screens.[57]

The burden and implications of HCV in thoracic solid organ transplant candidates are not well-characterized. Some studies suggest that the prevalence of HCV in thoracic solid organ transplants approximates that of the general population.[58] The impact of HCV on outcomes following solid organ transplantation has been studied extensively in renal transplantation, with HCV infection portending a poorer prognosis on overall patient and graft survival.[59,60]

There are scant data surrounding the impact of HCV on outcomes following HT, and recipient HCV seropositivity represents a relative contraindication to HT at many transplant centers. After HT, immunosuppressive medications may result in reactivation of latent HCV. Following reactivation, an increase in hepatitis viral replication can result in a varied clinical presentation, ranging from a complete lack of symptoms to fulminant liver failure and death.[61] A study of 200 HCV-seropositive HT recipients demonstrated reduced survival when compared with HCV-negative recipients, although this was not statistically significant after other donor and recipient clinical parameters were taken into account. There was no significant difference in the number of episodes of acute rejection in the first year following HT.[62] Another retrospective cohort study of more than 400 HCV-positive HT recipients demonstrated a statistically significant reduction in survival when compared with HCV-negative recipients.[63]

Transplantation of a heart from an HCV-positive donor into an uninfected recipient commonly results in chronic HCV infection in the recipient. An older study found that 82% of recipients of donor HCV-positive hearts became HCV RNA positive, with 30% ultimately developing HCV-related liver disease.[64] However, because of the immunocompromised state of the transplant recipient, anti-HCV antibodies may be undetectable in a large fraction of these patients.[64–66] Moreover, and also as a consequence of chronic immunosuppression, these patients may experience a significant delay between LFT elevation and the eventual detection of anti-HCV antibodies.[67] Although the impact of HCV donor positivity on mortality following HT is unclear, at least one multicenter study has suggested higher long-term mortality. These recipients were more likely to die of liver disease and allograft vasculopathy.[58]

The definition of "increased-risk" donors was originally put forth in the 1994 Public Health Service (PHS) guidelines and has since been expanded by many organ procurement organizations to include HCV.[68] Although the true prevalence of PHS-designated "increased-risk" donor hearts is unknown (as is the percentage of these hearts that originate from HCV-positive donors, and the subsequent rates of donor-to-recipient HCV transmission), the formal recommendation at many transplant centers is to decline donors with positive HCV NAT.[69]

According to the most recent Centers for Disease Control and Prevention guidelines, "Posttransplant HCV testing of recipients should be conducted when the donor (living or deceased) meets any of the following conditions: (1) identified as being at increased risk for HCV infection, (2) screening specimens are hemodiluted, (3) the medical/behavioral history is unavailable, or (4) the donor is infected with HCV. Recipient testing should be performed sometime between one and 3 months posttransplant to include HCV NAT (unless infection was documented pretransplant). NAT is important for HCV detection as infected recipients may remain Ab-negative due to immunosuppression."[69]

Novel agents for the treatment of hepatitis C virus and their implications for advanced therapies

Given the remarkable success of DAAs, the question of whether chronic HCV infection truly represents a contraindication to MCS or HT may be revisited. Ostensibly, advanced HF patients with chronic HCV could be treated with any of the aforementioned algorithms before or after undergoing MCS implantation or HT. In fact, in the International Society for Heart and Lung Transplantation's most recent listing criteria for HT, the organization states, "[t]he high level of anti-viral efficacy, acceptable safety profile, and expected less interaction with immunosuppressive regimens of direct-acting antiviral drugs will change our view on chronic HCV infection and transplantation in the coming years."[70]

Data surrounding treatment of HCV in LVAD recipients are virtually nonexistent. In the post-HT setting, IFN-based antiviral therapy has traditionally been avoided because it may increase the risk of allograft failure due to cardiotoxicity.[71] The European Association for the Study of the Liver cautions that because the risk of graft rejection on IFN-based treatment remains unclear, "treatment of chronic HCV infection in heart transplant recipients must be based on IFN-free regimens and the indication should be assessed on a case-by-case basis, if HCV infection is life-threatening."[72]

The American Association of Study of Liver Diseases and the Infectious Diseases Society of America have supported treatment of chronic HCV infection with DAAs in patients who have undergone solid organ transplantation.[73] Because of a shortage of deceased donor organs, the number of patients listed each year for HT routinely exceeds the number of patients actually undergoing transplantation. If the use of DAAs in the post-HT population continues to prove feasible and safe, the use of organs from HCV-positive donors may be an attractive option, because it may help to expand the donor pool to include HCV-positive organs for HCV-infected recipients. Drug-drug interactions between anti-HCV therapies and immunosuppressive medications have not been thoroughly investigated. Caution should be used with calcineurin inhibitors because of CYP3A4 interaction, and frequent monitoring should be used during DAA therapy post-HT.[74]

SUMMARY

Liver disease in the setting of advanced HF is common. Development of advanced fibrosis and cirrhosis due to chronic HF is often indolent, progressive, and difficult to diagnose despite maximal therapy. Identifying HF patients with severe hepatic fibrosis and cirrhosis before considering MCS and HT is critical, because these patients are at increased risk for morbidity and mortality. Further complicating the current understanding of cardiohepatic interactions in HF is the rising prevalence of HCV and evolving strategies for treatment. Based on current understanding, the authors propose the algorithm in **Fig. 4** to guide decision-making for advanced HF patients at high risk for chronic liver disease. Important to the care of HF patients with suspicion for cardiac liver disease and/or liver disease due to HCV is the inclusion of a multidisciplinary team comprising HF cardiology, hepatology, infectious disease, and pharmacy. There are gaps remaining in the understanding of cardiohepatic interactions in advanced HF that require ongoing investigation. However, a

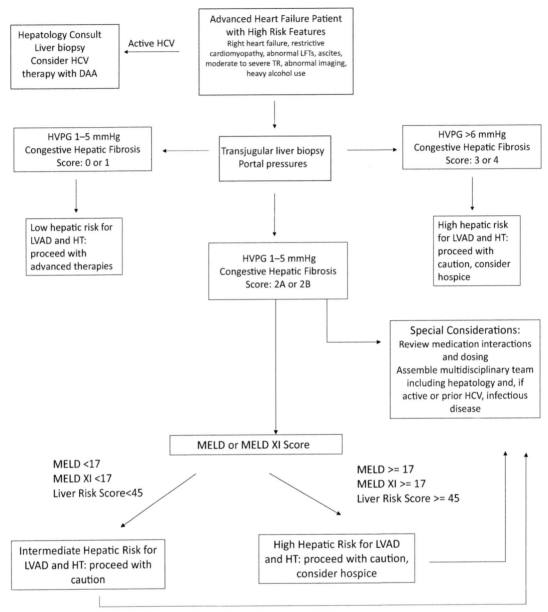

Fig. 4. Algorithm for the evaluation of liver disease in advanced HF patients.

thoughtful approach using clinical features, risk prediction tools, and histopathology can maximize outcomes for advanced HF patients in the current era of MCS and HT.

REFERENCES

1. Fang JC, Ewald GA, Allen LA, et al. Advanced (stage D) heart failure: a statement from the Heart Failure Society of America Guidelines Committee. J Card Fail 2015;21(6):519–34.
2. Nash K. Hepatology: clinical cases uncovered. Hoboken (NJ): Wiley-Blackwell; 2011. Available at: http://site.ebrary.com/lib/ohsu/reader.action?docID=10518665. Accessed Janruary 1, 2016.
3. Tapper EB, Sengupta N, Bonder A. The incidence and outcomes of ischemic hepatitis: a systematic review with meta-analysis. Am J Med 2015;128(12):1314–21.
4. Naschitz JE, Slobodin G, Lewis RJ, et al. Heart diseases affecting the liver and liver diseases affecting the heart. Am Heart J 2000;140(1):111–20.
5. Arcidi JM Jr, Moore GW, Hutchins GM. Hepatic morphology in cardiac dysfunction: a clinicopathologic study of 1000 subjects at autopsy. Am J Pathol 1981;104(2):159–66.

6. Henrion J, Schapira M, Luwaert R, et al. Hypoxic hepatitis: clinical and hemodynamic study in 142 consecutive cases. Medicine 2003;82(6):392–406.

7. Samsky MD, Patel CB, DeWald TA, et al. Cardiohepatic interactions in heart failure: an overview and clinical implications. J Am Coll Cardiol 2013; 61(24):2397–405.

8. Parola M, Robino G. Oxidative stress-related molecules and liver fibrosis. J Hepatol 2001;35(2): 297–306.

9. Tilg H, Kaser A, Moschen AR. How to modulate inflammatory cytokines in liver diseases. Liver Int 2006;26(9):1029–39.

10. Wanless IR, Liu JJ, Butany J. Role of thrombosis in the pathogenesis of congestive hepatic fibrosis (cardiac cirrhosis). Hepatology 1995; 21(5):1232–7.

11. Givertz MM. Assessing the liver to predict outcomes in heart transplantation. J Heart Lung Transplant 2015;34(7):869–72.

12. Gelow JM, Desai AS, Hochberg CP, et al. Clinical predictors of hepatic fibrosis in chronic advanced heart failure. Circ Heart Fail 2010;3(1):59–64.

13. Myers RP, Cerini R, Sayegh R, et al. Cardiac hepatopathy: clinical, hemodynamic, and histologic characteristics and correlations. Hepatology 2003;37(2): 393–400.

14. Ambrosy AP, Vaduganathan M, Huffman MD, et al. Clinical course and predictive value of liver function tests in patients hospitalized for worsening heart failure with reduced ejection fraction: an analysis of the EVEREST trial. Eur J Heart Fail 2012;14(3): 302–11.

15. Nikolaou M, Parissis J, Yilmaz MB, et al. Liver function abnormalities, clinical profile, and outcome in acute decompensated heart failure. Eur Heart J 2013;34(10):742–9.

16. Scholfield M, Schabath MB, Guglin M. Longitudinal trends, hemodynamic profiles, and prognostic value of abnormal liver function tests in patients with acute decompensated heart failure: an analysis of the ESCAPE trial. J Card Fail 2014;20(7): 476–84.

17. van Deursen VM, Edwards C, Cotter G, et al. Liver function, in-hospital, and post-discharge clinical outcome in patients with acute heart failure—results from the relaxin for the treatment of patients with acute heart failure study. J Card Fail 2014;20(6):407–13.

18. Samsky MD, Dunning A, DeVore AD, et al. Liver function tests in patients with acute heart failure and associated outcomes: insights from ASCEND-HF. Eur J Heart Fail 2015. [Epub ahead of print].

19. Lau GT, Tan HC, Kritharides L. Type of liver dysfunction in heart failure and its relation to the severity of tricuspid regurgitation. Am J Cardiol 2002;90(12): 1405–9.

20. van Deursen VM, Damman K, Hillege HL, et al. Abnormal liver function in relation to hemodynamic profile in heart failure patients. J Card Fail 2010; 16(1):84–90.

21. Bonekamp S, Kamel I, Solga S, et al. Can imaging modalities diagnose and stage hepatic fibrosis and cirrhosis accurately? J Hepatol 2009;50(1):17–35.

22. Kalambokis G, Manousou P, Vibhakorn S, et al. Transjugular liver biopsy–indications, adequacy, quality of specimens, and complications–a systematic review. J Hepatol 2007;47(2):284–94.

23. Groszmann RJ, Wongcharatrawee S. The hepatic venous pressure gradient: anything worth doing should be done right. Hepatology 2004;39(2):280–2.

24. Dai DF, Swanson PE, Krieger EV, et al. Congestive hepatic fibrosis score: a novel histologic assessment of clinical severity. Mod Pathol 2014;27(12): 1552–8.

25. Kim MS, Kato TS, Farr M, et al. Hepatic dysfunction in ambulatory patients with heart failure: application of the MELD scoring system for outcome prediction. J Am Coll Cardiol 2013;61(22):2253–61.

26. Abe S, Yoshihisa A, Takiguchi M, et al. Liver dysfunction assessed by model for end-stage liver disease excluding INR (MELD-XI) scoring system predicts adverse prognosis in heart failure. PLoS One 2014;9(6):e100618.

27. Lauer GM, Walker BD. Hepatitis C virus infection. N Engl J Med 2001;345(1):41–52.

28. Pawlotsky JM. Pathophysiology of hepatitis C virus infection and related liver disease. Trends Microbiol 2004;12(2):96–102.

29. Mailliard ME, Capadano ME, Hrnicek MJ, et al. Outcomes of a patient-to-patient outbreak of genotype 3a hepatitis C. Hepatology 2009;50(2):361–8.

30. Butt AA, Xiaoqiang W, Budoff M, et al. Hepatitis C virus infection and the risk of coronary disease. Clin Infect Dis 2009;49(2):225–32.

31. McKibben RA, Haberlen SA, Post WS, et al. A cross-sectional study of the association between chronic hepatitis C virus infection and subclinical coronary atherosclerosis among participants in the multicenter AIDS Cohort Study. J Infect Dis 2016; 213(2):257–65.

32. Matsumori A, Matoba Y, Sasayama S. Dilated cardiomyopathy associated with hepatitis C virus infection. Circulation 1995;92(9):2519–25.

33. Matsumori A, Shimada T, Chapman NM, et al. Myocarditis and heart failure associated with hepatitis C virus infection. J Card Fail 2006;12(4):293–8.

34. Sonnenblick M, Rosin A. Cardiotoxicity of interferon. A review of 44 cases. Chest 1991;99(3):557–61.

35. Afdhal N, Zeuzem S, Kwo P, et al. Ledipasvir and sofosbuvir for untreated HCV genotype 1 infection. N Engl J Med 2014;370(20):1889–98.

36. Kowdley KV, Gordon SC, Reddy KR, et al. Ledipasvir and sofosbuvir for 8 or 12 weeks for chronic

HCV without cirrhosis. N Engl J Med 2014;370(20): 1879–88.

37. FDA. FDA drug safety communication: FDA warns of serious slowing of the heart rate when antiarrhythmic drug amiodarone is used with hepatitis C treatments containing sofosbuvir (Harvoni) or Sovaldi in combination with another direct acting antiviral drug. 2015. Available at: http://www.fda.gov/Drugs/Drug Safety/ucm439484.htm. Accessed January 11, 2016.

38. Menon RM, Badri PS, Wang T, et al. Drug-drug interaction profile of the all-oral anti-hepatitis C virus regimen of paritaprevir/ritonavir, ombitasvir, and dasabuvir. J Hepatol 2015;63(1):20–9.

39. Matthews JC, Pagani FD, Haft JW, et al. Model for end-stage liver disease score predicts left ventricular assist device operative transfusion requirements, morbidity, and mortality. Circulation 2010;121(2): 214–20.

40. Yang JA, Kato TS, Shulman BP, et al. Liver dysfunction as a predictor of outcomes in patients with advanced heart failure requiring ventricular assist device support: use of the Model of End-stage Liver Disease (MELD) and MELD eXcluding INR (MELD-XI) scoring system. J Heart Lung Transplant 2012; 31(6):601–10.

41. Yost GL, Coyle L, Bhat G, et al. Model for end-stage liver disease predicts right ventricular failure in patients with left ventricular assist devices. J Artif Organs 2016;19(1):21–8.

42. Kim B, Tan A, Limketkai BN, et al. Comparison of outcome in patients with versus without ascites referred for either cardiac transplantation or ventricular assist device placement. Am J Cardiol 2015; 116(10):1596–600.

43. Reinhartz O, Farrar DJ, Hershon JH, et al. Importance of preoperative liver function as a predictor of survival in patients supported with Thoratec ventricular assist devices as a bridge to transplantation. J Thorac Cardiovasc Surg 1998;116(4):633–40.

44. Demirozu ZT, Hernandez R, Mallidi HR, et al. Heart-Mate II left ventricular assist device implantation in patients with advanced hepatic dysfunction. J Card Surg 2014;29(3):419–23.

45. Sargent JE, Dardas TF, Smith JW, et al. Periportal fibrosis without cirrhosis does not affect outcomes after continuous flow ventricular assist device implantation. J Thorac Cardiovasc Surg 2016;151(1): 230–5.

46. Farr M, Mitchell J, Lippel M, et al. Combination of liver biopsy with MELD-XI scores for post-transplant outcome prediction in patients with advanced heart failure and suspected liver dysfunction. J Heart Lung Transplant 2015;34(7):873–82.

47. Hsu RB, Lin FY, Chou NK, et al. Heart transplantation in patients with extreme right ventricular failure. Eur J Cardiothorac Surg 2007;32(3):457–61.

48. Hsu RB, Chang CI, Lin FY, et al. Heart transplantation in patients with liver cirrhosis. Eur J Cardiothorac Surg 2008;34(2):307–12.

49. Chokshi A, Cheema FH, Schaefle KJ, et al. Hepatic dysfunction and survival after orthotopic heart transplantation: application of the MELD scoring system for outcome prediction. J Heart Lung Transplant 2012;31(6):591–600.

50. Deo SV, Al-Kindi SG, Altarabsheh SE, et al. Model for end-stage liver disease excluding international normalized ratio (MELD-XI) score predicts heart transplant outcomes: evidence from the registry of the United Network for Organ Sharing. J Heart Lung Transplant 2016;35(2):222–7.

51. Louie CY, Pham MX, Daugherty TJ, et al. The liver in heart failure: a biopsy and explant series of the histopathologic and laboratory findings with a particular focus on pre-cardiac transplant evaluation. Mod Pathol 2015;28(7):932–43.

52. Cannon RM, Hughes MG, Jones CM, et al. A review of the United States experience with combined heart-liver transplantation. Transpl Int 2012;25(12): 1223–8.

53. Rana A, Robles S, Russo MJ, et al. The combined organ effect: protection against rejection? Ann Surg 2008;248(5):871–9.

54. Nelson LM, Penninga L, Sander K, et al. Long-term outcome in patients treated with combined heart and liver transplantation for familial amyloidotic cardiomyopathy. Clin Transplant 2013;27(2):203–9.

55. Rajagopalan N, Hoopes CW, Rosenau J. Hepatitis C virus infection in heart transplantation: is ventricular assist device therapy an option? Transplantation 2013;96(4):e23–4.

56. Meyer AL, Malehsa D, Budde U, et al. Acquired von Willebrand syndrome in patients with a centrifugal or axial continuous flow left ventricular assist device. JACC Heart Failure 2014;2(2):141–5.

57. Srivastava AV, Hrobowski T, Krese L, et al. High rates of false-positive hepatitis C antibody tests can occur after left ventricular assist device implantation. ASAIO J 2013;59(6):660–1.

58. Gasink LB, Blumberg EA, Localio AR, et al. Hepatitis C virus seropositivity in organ donors and survival in heart transplant recipients. JAMA 2006;296(15): 1843–50.

59. Romero E, Galindo P, Bravo JA, et al. Hepatitis C virus infection after renal transplantation. Transplant Proc 2008;40(9):2933–5.

60. González-Roncero F, Gentil MA, Valdivia MA, et al. Outcome of kidney transplant in chronic hepatitis C virus patients: effect of pretransplantation interferon-alpha2b monotherapy. Transplant Proc 2003;35(5):1745–7.

61. Roche B, Samuel D. The difficulties of managing severe hepatitis B virus reactivation. Liver Int 2011; 31(Suppl 1):104–10.

62. Fong TL, Hou L, Hutchinson IV, et al. Impact of hepatitis C infection on outcomes after heart transplantation. Transplantation 2009;88(9):1137–41.

63. Lee I, Localio R, Brensinger CM, et al. Decreased post-transplant survival among heart transplant recipients with pre-transplant hepatitis C virus positivity. J Heart Lung Transplant 2011;30:1266–74.

64. Ong JP, Barnes DS, Younossi ZM, et al. Outcome of de novo hepatitis C virus infection in heart transplant recipients. Hepatology 1999;30(5):1293–8.

65. Pfau PR, Rho R, DeNofrio D, et al. Hepatitis C transmission and infection by orthotopic heart transplantation. J Heart Lung Transplant 2000;19(4):350–4.

66. Zein NN, McGreger CG, Wendt NK, et al. Prevalence and outcome of hepatitis C infection among heart transplant recipients. J Heart Lung Transplant 1995;14(5):865–9.

67. Lunel F, Cadranel JF, Rosenheim M, et al. Hepatitis virus infections in heart transplant recipients: epidemiology, natural history, characteristics, and impact on survival. Gastroenterology 2000;119(4):1064–74.

68. Guidelines for preventing transmission of human immunodeficiency virus through transplantation of human tissue and organs. Centers for Disease Control and Prevention. MMWR Recomm Rep 1994;43(Rr-8):1–17.

69. Seem DL, Lee I, Umscheid CA, et al. PHS guideline for reducing human immunodeficiency virus, hepatitis B virus, and hepatitis C virus transmission through organ transplantation. Public Health Rep 2013;128(4):247–343.

70. Mehra MR, Canter CE, Hannan MM, et al. The 2016 International Society for Heart Lung Transplantation listing criteria for heart transplantation: a 10-year update. J Heart Lung Transplant 2016;35(1):1–23.

71. Kim E, Ko HH, Yoshida EM. A concise review of hepatitis C in heart and lung transplantation. Can J Gastroenterol 2011;25(8):445–8.

72. EASL Recommendations on Treatment of Hepatitis C 2015. J Hepatol 2015;63(1):199–236.

73. AASLD-IDSA. Recommendations for testing, managing, and treating hepatitis C. 2015. Available at: http://www.hcvguidelines.org. Accessed January 14, 2016.

74. Hulskotte E, Gupta S, Xuan F, et al. Pharmacokinetic interaction between the hepatitis C virus protease inhibitor boceprevir and cyclosporine and tacrolimus in healthy volunteers. Hepatology 2012; 56(5):1622–30.

Frailty in Advanced Heart Failure

Emer Joyce, MD, PhD

KEYWORDS

- Frailty • Advanced heart failure • Sarcopenia • Cachexia • Fried phenotype
- Left ventricular assist device

KEY POINTS

- Frailty and associated conditions (cachexia, sarcopenia) are highly prevalent in patients with advanced heart failure (HF), and both syndromes share common underlying pathobiological processes.
- Frailty is associated with worse outcomes after interventional therapies (including mechanical circulatory support and heart transplantation), defines risk not yet captured by traditional risk scores, and represents a useful incremental prognostic tool to aid patient selection for advanced therapies.
- There is an unmet need for a single validated tool or scale capable of accurately defining frailty in the advanced HF population and is responsive to positive interventions.
- Left ventricular assist device implantation may be able to "de-frail" patients with predominantly HF-related (in contrast to age- or comorbidity-related) frailty by reversing myocardial failure and restoring cardiac output.

INTRODUCTION

Frailty is formally defined as a biologic syndrome reflecting a state of impaired physiologic and homeostatic reserve and heightened vulnerability to stressors, resulting from the accumulation of multiple morbidities, aging, and disability.[1,2] The evolving profile of cardiovascular disease, increased survival of aging patients with complex comorbidities, in parallel with an ever-expanding array of invasive therapeutic interventions, means that cardiologists (and, in particular, heart failure [HF] specialists) are becomingly increasingly aware of the burden of frailty and its downstream consequences on postintervention outcomes in their patients. Older patients with HF have consistently demonstrated the highest prevalence of frailty, up to 50% in some studies.[2,3] The strong association between HF and frailty is particularly

evident in the setting of advanced HF, wherein the frail phenotype and associated cachexia and generalized muscle weakness frequently manifest in the later stages of disease. Although increasingly prevalent with advancing age, advanced age is not a prerequisite for frailty, with end-stage HF being a clinical prototype for "age-independent" frailty. In one study of 622 patients referred to an HF unit, one-third of patients less than the age of 70 years fulfilled one or more pre-specified criteria for frailty.[4] This close overlap between both syndromes is particularly relevant in the setting of advanced HF patients being considered for high-risk invasive therapies, including left ventricular assist device implantation (LVAD) and/or cardiac transplantation.

Despite varying modes of assessment of frailty and variability in incorporated domains (biological, nutritional, functional, and cognitive), almost every

Disclosure Statement: The author has nothing to disclose.
Section of Heart Failure and Cardiac Transplant Medicine, Robert and Suzanne Tomsich Department of Cardiovascular Medicine, Sydell and Arnold Miller Family Heart and Vascular Institute, Cleveland Clinic Foundation, 9500 Euclid Avenue, J3-4, Cleveland, OH 44195, USA
E-mail address: joycee@ccf.org

heartfailure.theclinics.com

proposed single- or multi-item definition has been associated with, or shown to be predictive of, adverse outcome in cardiovascular disease populations, including HF patients.[2] Frailty assessment therefore appears to contribute valuable and incremental prognostic insights in HF. The aim of this review is to focus on the role of frailty in advanced HF patients, including its prevalence, impact on morbidity and mortality, potential for refining candidate selection for advanced therapies, and in certain cases, possibility for regression following the restoration of cardiac output inherent with LVAD and/or cardiac transplantation.

PATHOBIOLOGY OF FRAILTY IN ADVANCED HEART FAILURE

The cycle of frailty, as hypothesized by Fried and colleagues,[1] is initiated by disease- and/or aging-related declines in lean muscle mass and strength, leading to reduced activity level and walking speed, and in turn, ultimately leading to and further compounded by weight loss and malnutrition. Considerable overlap exists in the constellation of weakness, wasting, exercise intolerance, and exhaustion that can manifest in both progressive HF and frailty (Fig. 1). Because of the fact that each syndrome may mimic the other, objective tools are needed to provide an independent assessment of the presence and severity of the frail phenotype in HF patients. The need for objective tools is even more important in advanced HF patients, where worsening fatigue, declining physical activity, and cachexia may reflect progressive myocardial failure and related downstream multiorgan system dysfunction requiring evaluation of candidacy for end-stage disease management options rather than

a distinct frailty substrate predominantly driven by aging and other comorbidities.

The degree of clinical similarity between frailty and chronic HF reflects the many common pathobiological processes across multiple physiologic systems (including immunologic, metabolic, neurohormonal, and autonomic-based domains) shared by both syndromes. Each syndrome in turn increases risk for development of[5,6] and potentiates increasing morbidity[7–10] in the other, likely as a result of this common pathophysiologic pathway. Sarcopenia represents a key component of the frailty syndrome and is defined as a progressive loss of muscle mass and strength, beyond that expected from normal aging.[11] Intrinsic histologic and biochemical skeletal muscle changes, including fiber atrophy, increased type IIb fibers, and decreased oxidative capacity, are also characteristic of symptomatic HF.[12] Cachexia is a related condition that is incorporated as 1 of the 5 key domains in the traditional frail phenotype model.[1] It is also commonly used to describe the muscle wasting and tissue loss seen in advanced stages of HF and is formally defined as loss of greater than 5% of total body weight over the preceding 6 months.[13]

Inflammatory biomarkers (including interleukin-1, interleukin-6, tumor necrosis factor-α, and C-reactive protein) known to underpin disease development and progression in chronic HF by contributing to tissue wasting and cardiac cachexia[14] have also been demonstrated as biologic mediators of the frailty phenotype.[15,16] Dysregulated neurohormonal mechanisms, including those involving cortisol regulation and the growth hormone/insulin-like growth factor-1 (GH/IGF-1) signaling axis, leading to downstream anabolic-catabolic uncoupling and resultant

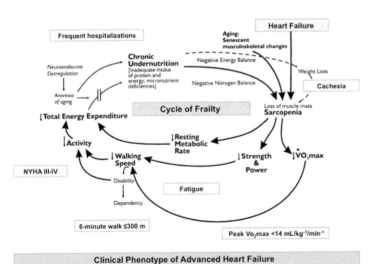

Fig. 1. Overlap between the clinical phenotypes of frailty and advanced HF. Elements of the classic cycle of frailty may also reflect key clinical markers in the progression of advanced HF. (Adapted from Fried LP, Tangen CM, Walston J, et al. Frailty in older adults: evidence for a phenotype. J Gerontol A Biol Sci Med Sci 2001;56:M147; with permission.)

muscle wasting, have also been implicated in both disease states.[17–21] This enhanced catabolic milieu has been significantly associated with objective disease severity in chronic HF as measured by symptom-limited cardiopulmonary exercise testing, with higher levels of cortisol predicting more impaired peak VO_2, worse ventilatory inefficiency, and chronotropic incompetence.[22]

In summary, frailty is a syndrome characterized by a global imbalance between an anabolic and catabolic state, leading to muscle wasting and loss (sarcopenia), and eventually, to cachexia. Progressive HF is characterized not only by myocardial but also by metabolic failure[23] and thus shares many of these cellular and molecular consequences, although the exact mechanisms of HF-specific frailty have yet to be determined.

ASSESSMENT OF FRAILTY IN ADVANCED HEART FAILURE

Multiple measures have been developed to define frailty, largely focusing on 1 or more of the 5 core domains of the phenotype: shrinking, weakness, exhaustion, slowness, and inactivity.[2] The Fried scale, also known as the frail phenotype, is the most extensively validated and frequently cited assessment tool across all cardiovascular populations (**Box 1**).[1,2] To date, no specific definition has been validated for frailty assessment in any HF population. Selecting the most appropriate measurement tool is essential, given that different approaches may identify different subsets of patients with only limited overlap.[24] Those measures that have been studied in advanced HF patients include the Fried scale,[1] the deficit index,[9,25] and single-item components of the Fried scale, particularly grip strength.[10,26]

The "deficit index" is a composite measure calculated by summing impairments in activities of daily living, comorbid conditions, and abnormal laboratory values.[25] The higher the index, the more likely patients are frail, thereby allowing some degree of quantification of the severity as well as the absolute presence of frailty. However, the long list of variables needed for screening makes it cumbersome and unsuitable for more urgent situations. Single-item measures rather than multicomponent scales have several advantages, including their practicality and potential for increased feasibility in more limited populations, including advanced HF patients being assessed for advanced therapies. Hand grip strength, easily and quickly measured using a simple hand-held device, appears especially suitable for hospitalized and immobile HF patients and has already been tested in the LVAD population.[10,26] Although

---

Box 1
Fried scale

1. *Shrinking*: Unintentional weight loss
   a. $\geq$10 lbs or $\geq$5% of total body weight in past year
2. *Weakness*: Reduced hand grip strength
   a. Lowest quintile according to gender/body mass index, as measured by a hand dynamometer
      i. Maximum isometric contraction in dominant hand over 3 attempts
3. *Exhaustion*: Self-reported exhaustion
   a. $\geq$3 days answered to 2 questions from Center for Epideimological Studies–Depression scale
      i. How often in the past week did you feel like everything was an effort?
      ii. How often in the past week did you feel like you could not get going?
4. *Slowness:* Slow gait speed
   a. Slowest quintile according to gender/height based on time to walk 15 feet
5. *Inactivity*: Low self-reported physical activity
   a. Lowest quintile of kilocalories (kcal) expended per week based on a questionnaire that links kilocalorie expenditure to activity level
      i. Men: positive if <383 kcal/wk
      ii. Women: positive if <270 kcal/wk

Frail $\geq$3 criteria present

Intermediate/Prefrail: 1 or 2 criteria present

Advantages

- Extensively validated
- Has predicted both morbidity and mortality in large community-dwelling cohorts of cardiovascular disease patients
- Relative ease of implementation

Disadvantages

- May not be feasible or useful in more debilitated HF populations such as those who cannot ambulate, so-called floor effect
- Does not incorporate the domains of cognition, mood, and nutrition

Data from Fried LP, Tangen CM, Walston J, et al. Frailty in older adults: evidence for a phenotype. J Gerontol A Biol Sci Med Sci 2001;56:M146–56.

not systematically studied yet in the advanced HF population, gait speed has also amassed a robust evidence base as a frailty-proxy in other cardiovascular and cardiac surgical settings[2] and could also be conceivably incorporated into the clinical assessment of all ambulatory end-stage HF patients.

Ultimately, heterogeneity in patient profiles can preclude recommendation of a single approach or tool. Different aspects of the clinical frail phenotype may either dominate or be entirely absent in the same patient. Advanced HF induces age-independent biological frailty, which has implications for modes of assessment based on predominantly geriatric domains. In a study of 360 all-comer HF patients treated in a multidisciplinary HF unit, activity level and cognitive function were impaired more frequently in older (≥70 years) patients, as expected, while depressive symptoms were found to be equally as prevalent in younger and older HF patients, highlighting the importance of considering mood evaluation as an important component of the phenotype in this cohort.[6] Moreover, not all variables may influence outcomes to the same degree, and weighting of certain factors in disease-specific risk scores may ultimately be required. In advanced stage D HF patients, the degree of debilitation associated with hemodynamic insufficiency may induce a floor effect, where administered tools may record lowest possible values, or may not be feasible at all. For these patients, determining which aspects of the individual's frail substrate may be treatment-responsive versus nonresponsive alongside establishing that the overall burden of frailty may be equally as important, given the implications for determining viable candidacy for advanced therapies, discussed in more detail later. Overall, optimal tools to define, quantify, and monitor frailty and its related domains in HF patients, and in particular advanced HF patients, remain a relevant area of unmet need.[27]

ROLE FOR FRAILTY ASSESSMENT IN ADVANCED HEART FAILURE

Surgical therapies for advanced HF represent a highly clinical relevant arena in which to assess upfront the potential for adverse downstream effects of both the presence and the severity of component aspects of the frail phenotype (tissue loss, cognitive deficits) as well as its potential impact on early (periprocedural) and later (survival beyond 1 year) outcomes. Frailty in elderly populations undergoing cardiac surgery has already been definitively related to adverse outcomes, including postoperative morbidity and increased

mortality.[28,29] Conversely, this consistent marker of increased risk is not yet captured by traditional surgical risk scores.[29] In a study of 131 elderly patients undergoing coronary artery bypass and/or valve surgery, slow gait speed conferred a 2- to 3-fold increased risk of in-hospital mortality or major morbidity for any given level of Society of Thoracic Surgeons score; adjusted odds ratio was 3.05.[29]

Destination therapy (DT) LVAD is a particularly compelling setting for determining the presence of frailty, given that by definition, these patients are typically of advancing age and/or possess a significant noncardiac comorbidity profile, which renders them ineligible for cardiac transplantation, but should still have reasonable life expectancy and residual quality of life postprocedure to be able to realize the benefits of the device. Morbidity and mortality remain significant issues following LVAD implantation,[30] and therefore, appropriate patient selection continues to be of paramount importance in ensuring favorable outcomes. Existing risk prediction models for postdevice outcomes have shown very limited discrimination,[31] and, as in other cardiac surgery procedures, have not formally incorporated frailty measures. In addition, the frail phenotype or related sarcopenia and/or cachexia have not yet been investigated as independent markers of adverse post-LVAD outcome in the annual Interagency Registry for Mechanically Assisted Circulatory Support (INTERMACS) reports.[32] Notably, 30% of LVAD implants (n = 9000) between 2008 and 2013 occurred in patients older than the age of 65.[32] Although older age has been associated with a worse prognosis in clinical trials of the HeartMate II device in both bridge-to-transplant and DT populations,[31] other single-center studies have conversely shown comparable survival, and importantly, improvement in functional capacity and quality of life, in LVAD recipients older than 70 years of age compared with those less than 70 years of age.[33] This finding underlines that fact that just as advancing age does not directly equate to frailty, frailty in HF does not directly equate to advanced age. Applying objective measures to assess frailty in this population is an obvious adjunctive risk stratification tool to provide clearer distinction between a potential DT-LVAD candidate's chronologic versus biological fingerprint.

In parallel with the rising use of mechanical circulatory support devices as lifelong therapy in older patients with multimorbidity, an increasing proportion of older, otherwise eligible end-stage HF patients are being referred for heart transplantation; more than 1% of cardiac transplants are now performed in patients older than 70 years of age.[34] Increasing recipient age is associated with higher posttransplant mortality and morbidity.[34] Given the association of frailty with both advancing age and advancing HF, and the demonstration of poorer outcomes in frail older patients undergoing cardiac surgery,[28,29] it is clear that looking for (and potentially intervening on) frailty in this evolving heart transplant population should also be a clinical priority.

PREVALENCE AND IMPACT OF FRAILTY IN ADVANCED HEART FAILURE

Published studies evaluating the prevalence of frailty and its association with outcome in advanced HF populations are outlined in **Table 1**. Although the most person-years accrued for studies of frailty in cardiovascular disease are for HF,[2] applying measures of frailty as an adjunctive prognostic tool in the care of stage D HF patients is an emerging field. Studies in stage C patients have consistently shown increased risk for hospitalizations, higher mortality, and impaired quality of life in those meeting criteria for frailty.[4,7,35] In a more symptomatic and progressed HF population undergoing cardiac resynchronization therapy, 28% of patients met criteria for frailty, as defined by the Fried scale.[8] Despite successful device implantation, frail patients were more likely to experience subsequent episodes of decompensated HF over 12 months of follow-up.[8]

The study by Dunlay and colleagues[9] marks the first significant investigation focusing on the burden of frailty, as measured by the deficit index, and its impact in the DT-LVAD population. Using the standard definition of frailty according to this multiparametric tool, almost 62% of this population (n = 99) would be considered frail; to allow for obvious differences unique to this cohort of patients for this analysis, those in the highest tertile were considered frail. Importantly, patients defined as frail at the time of LVAD implantation had a 3-fold increased risk of death during follow-up and an almost 1.5 times increased risk of rehospitalization, independent of age, gender, and INTERMACS profile.[9] One-year postimplant death rates for frail patients approached 40%, whereas nonfrail patients showed a 1-year mortality (16.2%) in line with expected INTERMACS estimates. Given that the deficit index provides a fairly rigorous and incremental assessment of an individual's frail substrate, it is not surprising that rehospitalizations were more prevalent in this group. However, it was notable that these readmissions were for typical post-LVAD reasons: gastrointestinal bleeding, ventricular arrhythmias,

and HF, rather than seemingly more direct frailty-mediated causes like recurrent falls or systemic infections. It is possible that cognitive decline and lack of independence taking prescribed medication, included as component parts of the index, may be playing a more indirect, intermediary role (such as difficulty getting to laboratory appointments leading to supratherapeutic anticoagulation and bleeding, missing antiarrhythmic/diuretic) in these presentations than previously thought. Overall, frail patients were found to spend an average of 6 additional weeks in the hospital in their first year after LVAD compared with their nonfrail counterparts, underlying the importance of considering the identification and scope of the burden of frailty in these patients for health care utilization and resource planning, in addition to harder endpoints, in this population.

In the absence of an accepted gold-standard tool, an alternative approach to characterizing frailty in potential LVAD candidates is to evaluate the diagnostic accuracy and predictive capabilities of a single screening measure that serves as representative of a key component of the phenotype. Chung and colleagues[10] used hand grip strength as an index of skeletal myopathy in 72 patients pre-LVAD implantation and subsequently recorded early postoperative morbidity and survival up to 3 years of follow-up. Weak grip strength, defined as less than 25% of total body weight, was present in more than one-fifth (22%) of the cohort. This relatively high prevalence is especially notable given the younger age of this population, mean age 59 ± 2 years, most likely reflecting a mixed-strategy device group, but nonetheless further underlining that when it comes to advanced HF, frailty does not require advancing age as a cofactor. Those patients with weak grip strength went on to suffer reduced survival after LVAD as well as higher postoperative complication rates (bleeding and infection) compared with those with normal grip strength, although it is important to note event rates between groups were not adjusted for age or INTERMACS profile. This study highlights that even single-item measures of skeletal muscle function, probably through identifying the sarcopenic substrate of frailty, can provide prognostic value in this population. Interestingly, there were no differences in baseline clinical, biochemical, or hemodynamic parameters between weak or normal grip strength groups, suggesting that grip strength does indeed identify additional risk not yet being measured by conventional variables. Grip strength as a marker of frailty has been validated as an independent predictor of adverse outcomes in many diverse populations.[27,36] Its particular advantage over other

Table 1
Published studies evaluating frailty in advanced heart failure populations

Author, y	N	Patient Population	Frailty Tool	Prevalence of Frailty	Outcome(s) for Frail vs Nonfrail
Dominguez-Rodriguez et al,[8] 2015	102	NYHA III–IV LVEF <30% Age ≥70 y Nonischemic Undergoing CRT-D	Fried scale ≥3	28% (n = 29)	1-y risk of acute decompensated HF: 56% vs 16%; HR 4.55, 95% CI 1.7–12.0
Jha et al,[37] 2016	120	NYHA III–IV Mean LVEF 27% ± 14% Age 53 ± 12 y Referred for and/or listed for heart transplantation	Fried scale ≥3	33% (n = 39)	1-y actuarial survival: 54% ± 9% vs 79% ± 5%, P<.005 1-y BTT-LVAD and transplant-free survival: 58% ± 12% vs 78% ± 6%, P<.05
Chung et al,[10] 2014	72	NYHA III–IV Mean LVEF 17.9% ± 0.6% Age 59 ± 2 y Undergoing LVAD	Grip strength Weak if <25% total body weight	22% (n = 16)	6-mo survival: 75% vs 93%, log rank 0.02 Postoperative bleeding: 54% vs 17%, P = .002 Postoperative infection: 85 vs 54, P = .01
Dunlay et al,[9] 2014	99	INTERMACS profile 4 (IQR 3,5) Mean LVEF 18.5% ± 6.8% Age 65 ± 9 y Undergoing LVAD	Deficit index Frail if >32% deficits (lower tertile)	34% (n = 33) 62% by standard definition[45]	1-y all-cause mortality: adjusted[a] HR 3.08, 95% CI 1.2–5.0 Rehospitalizations (1.9 ± 1.6 y mean follow-up): adjusted[a] HR 1.42, 95% CI 0.98–2.1 Days alive outside of hospital at 1 y: 250 vs 293
Khawaja et al,[26] 2014	15	Age 62 ± 7 y Undergoing LVAD vs 10 controls (no cardiac disease, nonsmokers)	Grip strength	Mean grip strength 35.8 ± 7.8 vs 55.6 ± 12.7 kg (P = .001)	Change in grip strength at 6 mo on LVAD: +25.5% ± 27.5%

Abbreviations: BTT, bridge-to-transplant; CI, confidence interval; CRT-D, cardiac resynchronization therapy-defibrillator; HR, hazard ratio; IQR, interquartile range; LVEF, left ventricular ejection fraction.
[a] Adjusted for age, gender, INTERMACS profile.

easily administered single-item measures such as gait speed is that it can also be performed in wheelchair- or bed-bound patients, making it accessible to almost all advanced HF patients.

It is important to note that both of these studies are limited by their smaller sample sizes, single-center setting, observational design, and lack of demonstration of incremental value of frailty assessment over traditional risk scores used to assess outcome after LVAD implantation, including the HeartMate II risk score.[31] Larger, multicenter collaborative studies are required to determine the true burden, nature, and severity of frailty in this patient subset, its impact on outcomes, and potential for modification. Subsequent studies in this population, particularly in the DT patients, should also focus on predicting patient-centered outcomes, such as return to independent living or quality of life, for which frailty has demonstrated promise in other cardiovascular domains. Based on currently available evidence, declining candidacy for advanced therapies based on frailty alone is not supported at the present time.

In the cardiac transplantation population, even less data are available regarding the prevalence and prognostic impact of frailty, despite recipient profiles also undergoing marked evolution over the past decade, most notably the increase in the number of patients of older age and greater comorbidity burden.[30] One recent study by Jha and colleagues[37] attempts to address this knowledge gap, providing assessment of frailty using a modified Fried scale, in addition to cognitive function and depression screening, in 120 patients referred for or listed for heart transplantation, with 34 patients ultimately undergoing transplant surgery included in the analysis. One-third of the total cohort, mean age of 53 ± 12 years, was classified as frail. Overall, being frail conferred a significantly reduced 1-year actuarial survival and 1-year bridge-to-transplant LVAD and heart transplant–free survival[37] (see **Table 1**). Frail patients who underwent transplantation (26%, n = 9) had a survival rate at 1 year of $52\% \pm 23\%$ versus 100% of nonfrail patients. In addition, they showed trends toward longer intensive care unit (median 8 vs 6 days) and total hospital stay (median 27 vs 24 days).[37] The study was not powered to determine the true difference in mortality rates between frail and nonfrail patients across such a heterogeneous cohort: patients referred but not listed, patients listed but subsequently dying on waiting list or after ventricular assist device (VAD) surgery, listed patients still waiting for transplant with or without LVAD in addition to patients actually undergoing transplantation. Nonetheless, the crude finding of almost a doubling in mortality in frail

compared with nonfrail patients initially considered potential candidates for cardiac transplantation is sobering and heralds the rather urgent need for more research in this domain. Notably, these patients did present as an overall worse HF subgroup: they were more symptomatic (New York Heart Association [NYHA] Class IV >>III) and displayed worse invasive hemodynamics (higher filling pressures, lower cardiac indices) and more adverse biochemical profiles (anemia, hypoalbuminemia, elevated bilirubin). This study seems to suggest in younger patients eligible for transplant that frailty is largely a function of HF severity. These findings could potentially offer optimism for its reversal following definitive treatment of the HF; optimism that is not borne out by the subsequent survival statistics, although the complexity of this "all-comer" population, heterogeneity, in ultimate treatment strategies and outside factors such as wait list time, prevent drawing any major conclusions from this single data set. These findings also appear to differ from the findings by Chung and colleagues[10] in a similar younger-age, mixed indication LVAD cohort. However, this likely reflects the differences in the methods used to define frailty across both studies: hand grip strength alone (specific for muscle weakness/wasting) versus the modified Fried phenotype used (inclusion of more nonspecific components that may overlap between the 2 syndromes such as exhaustion, low physical activity, reduced appetite).[10,37] Although frailty may be largely a function of advanced HF in younger patients referred for advanced therapies, by the time they have traveled through the stages of their HF trajectory, frailty accrued over time may be more "resistant" and not simply reversed by correcting underlying cardiac output failure. This study also highlights the need for future studies more reflective of the increasingly older-age cohort being considered for transplantation.

CONCEPT OF FRAILTY "REVERSAL" IN ADVANCED HEART FAILURE

The unique aspect of the study of frailty in advanced HF patients is that the HF itself and resultant end-organ dysfunction, clinical and subclinical, independent of age and associated age-activated pathobiological pathways, can simulate the phenotype. This simulation leads to the consideration of the degree to which HF-associated frailty may be potentially reversible with LVAD implantation, which of course has the potential to remove one of the principal underlying drivers of the frail phenotype, myocardial failure, in appropriate patients. The key step is identifying these potential "LVAD-sensitive" individuals upfront as part of the selection process. Flint and colleagues[27] proposed a model whereby patients being evaluated for DT-LVAD with a similar overall burden of frailty could be further subdivided into 3 broad groups: those with primarily "LVAD-responsive" frailty (direct consequence of the HF itself and thus potentially fully reversible); those with primarily "LVAD-independent" frailty (largely resulting from noncardiac conditions and thus most likely nonreversible with advanced therapies); and finally, those who have a significant component of HF-related frailty but also a significant burden of non-HF morbidity and/or advancing age disqualifying them from heart transplantation and likely contributing to their frailty (**Fig. 2**). It is

less clear in these "LVAD-intermediate" patients how responsive their frail substrate may be to the restoration of adequate cardiac output alone.

In an ideal scenario, frailty measures would be able to distinguish potential reversible from irreversible frailty, thereby enhancing clinicians' ability to identify those candidates most likely to not only survive but also to "survive well." This concept is supported by preliminary data from the aforementioned study of handgrip strength in LVAD patients,[10] whereby, in addition to preimplantation, hand grip strength was also serially measured in a small subset of patients (n = 27) following LVAD implantation. Throughout a 6-month follow-up period, grip strength increased consistently, and by 6 months, had increased by a

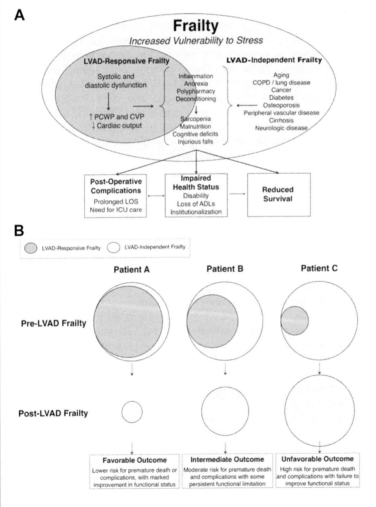

Fig. 2. (A) Breakdown of frailty into its underlying causes, manifestations, and clinical outcomes separated by LVAD-responsive and LVAD-independent causes of frailty. Frailty is a heightened state of vulnerability in the face of stress and results from the accumulation of multimorbidity, aging, and disability. In advanced HF with reduced left ventricular ejection fraction, a patient's HF contributes significantly to the frailty syndrome and is potentially reversible with LVAD (LVAD-responsive frailty). However, many patients with advanced HF may be frail due to illness unrelated to HF severity, which is not treatable with LVAD (LVAD-independent frailty). HF-related and non-HF-related factors combine to adversely affect health outcomes through several common effectors of frailty. (B) Patients undergoing DT-LVAD with similar total baseline frailty but differing underlying causes of frailty. Patient A, with primarily LVAD-responsive frailty (ie, mostly HF-related illness), is likely to experience a good outcome if he or she survives the early postoperative period. Conversely, Patient C, with primarily LVAD-independent frailty (ie, mostly noncardiac-related illness), is at greater risk of death, complications (eg, stroke, gastrointestinal bleed, or chronic hemolytic anemia), and/or persistently poor functional status after LVAD placement. Of note, most DT patients are more like Patient B, with evidence of significant LV dysfunction warranting LVAD but also significant comorbidity and/or advanced age disqualifying them from transplantation. ADLs, activities of daily living; CVP, central venous pressure; COPD, chronic obstructive pulmonary disease; ICU, intensive care unit; LOS, length of stay; PCWP, pulmonary capillary wedge pressure. (*From* Flint KM, Matlock DD, Lindenfeld J, et al. Frailty and the selection of patients for destination therapy left ventricular assist device. Circ Heart Fail 2012;5(2):289; with permission.)

mean of almost 50%.[10] Confirmation of the positive functional as well as cellular and molecular effects of LVAD support (mean 358 ± 294 days) and resultant restoration of cardiac output on muscle structure and metabolism was provided in a recent study of 31 advanced HF patients (mean age 62 ± 8 years) treated with LVAD implantation.[26] Rectus abdominis muscle samples at explant showed increased cross-sectional area of muscle fibers, relative increase of type 1 fibers, and a decreased proportion of type II fibers compared with biopsies taken at the time of implant, signifying improving oxidative capacity.[26] Notably also, GH/IGF-1 signaling axis had corrected, and hand-grip strength had increased by 26.5% ± 27.5% (P<.05 vs baseline) by the time of LVAD explant.[26] This study is small and preliminary, but nonetheless, provides exciting evidence that left-sided mechanical circulatory support may have the ability to positively modify, if not reverse, many of the adverse metabolic, neurohormonal, and functional impairments associated with HF-related frailty. A clinical trial is currently ongoing (NCT02156583) using the Fried scale as well as the Short Physical Performance Battery to assess change in clinical frailty at 6 months post-LVAD in patients 60 years of age and older undergoing HeartMate II implantation. Finally, LVAD support has also demonstrated a beneficial effect on cardiac cachexia and nutritional parameters in advanced HF patients; 75% of patients deemed underweight at the time of implant were found to show clinically meaningful weight gain at 24 months in a recent analysis of 896 patients enrolled across HeartMate II clinical trials.[38]

Although considered most relevant in the clinical setting of DT-LVAD support, the contemporary trend for listing older and more comorbid HF patients for cardiac transplantation means that distinction between HF-related frailty and that due to age- and other noncardiac-related illnesses is poised to become more important in the transplant-eligible population, particularly in light of both the sustained donor organ shortage and the inherent toxicities associated with immunosuppressive regimens in this population.

GENERAL STRATEGIES FOR MODIFICATION OF FRAILTY IN ADVANCED HEART FAILURE

Although the concept of reversibility of frailty remains controversial in those patients with advanced HF undergoing invasive therapies, several noninvasive interventions to improve or modify the phenotype have been studied in both general elderly populations and HF patients (**Box 2**). Frail HF patients appear to particularly

---

> **Box 2**
> **Studied interventions for frailty modification**
>
> - Specialized heart failure clinics/disease management programs[39]
> - Multidisciplinary interventions[42]
> - Geriatric consultation[46]
> - Exercise training[40,41,47,48]
> - Nutritional supplementation[47]
> - β-Blocker uptitration[49]
> - Testosterone replacement[50]
> - Polypharmacy reduction[51]

benefit from specialized HF disease management programs.[39] Exercise training has also proven its significant positive role in modifying both hard endpoints (mortality, HF-related hospitalizations) and patient-centered outcomes (health-related quality of life, depressive symptoms) in chronic HF patients, including patients with NYHA III–IV symptoms.[40,41] The Frailty Intervention Trial has recently shown successful improvement (14.7% at 12 months) in frailty parameters in a general population of elderly patients (n = 216, mean age 83 years) using specific, targeted multidisciplinary interventions for each component of the Fried scale.[42] Similar studies in advanced HF patients being considered for high-risk surgical therapies in order to determine if such interventions can positively modify the inflammatory, neurohormonal and metabolic aspects specific to the frailty substrate in this milieu are needed. The concept of "prehabilitation" has been explored in general surgical populations and is gaining traction but has not yet been studied in this cohort.[43] At the very least, in those selected for advanced therapies, defining the burden of frailty in individual patients upfront facilitates the identification of those patients who may warrant more aggressive rehabilitation and/or closer follow-up following their surgery. Finally, for patients with end-stage disease and associated marked disability as well as general frailty, early involvement of palliative and/or supportive care services should be considered.

SUMMARY AND FUTURE DIRECTIONS

Frailty is highly prevalent in patients with advanced HF and appears to provide prognostic information not captured by traditional risk assessment. As indications for the use of mechanical circulatory support have evolved and the population of patients undergoing LVAD implantation as lifelong therapy has grown larger, the adverse complication rate has remained static,[30] and thereby, it has become increasingly important to select optimal recipients with greatest likelihood of benefit. Incorporating frailty assessment as a novel tool in advanced therapy evaluation protocols may help determine the overall "net" gain, and not just the disease-specific gain, following a potentially high-risk procedure such as LVAD implantation in this high-risk patient group. A standardized definition of frailty validated for HF patients is the first important step and will better facilitate the design of therapeutic interventions along the HF disease continuum, ideally before their progression to stage D disease. A consensus statement outlining ongoing efforts to integrate both the phenotype and the deficit index models for a solid operational definition of frailty was recently released.[44] The possibility that surgical advanced therapies (VAD, cardiac transplantation) capable of reversing myocardial failure could potentially "de-frail" those patients with a greater proportion of HF-related rather than age- or comorbidity-related frailty is an exciting prospect but requires further prospective and ideally multicenter studies. It is likely that in some patients, individual components of the frail phenotype may not be created equally, and a more targeted approach to modify specific aspects such as cachexia or sarcopenia may be required. Regardless of the intervention, management of frail advanced HF patients should emphasize patient-centered outcomes including quality of life and functional status. Ultimately, improving the understanding of the close interactions between advanced HF, frailty, and aging should significantly help guide the frequently difficult clinical decision-making required in this complex patient group.

REFERENCES

1. Fried LP, Tangen CM, Walston J, et al. Frailty in older adults: evidence for a phenotype. J Gerontol A Biol Sci Med Sci 2001;56:M146–56.
2. Afilalo J, Alexander KP, Mack MJ, et al. Frailty assessment in the cardiovascular care of older adults. J Am Coll Cardiol 2014;63:747–62.
3. Murad K, Kitzman DW. Frailty and multiple comorbidities in the elderly patient with heart failure: implications for management. Heart Fail Rev 2012;17: 581–8.
4. Lupon J, Gonzalez B, Santaeugenia S, et al. Prognostic implication of frailty and depressive symptoms in an outpatient population with heart failure. Rev Esp Cardiol 2008;61:835–42.
5. Khan H, Kalogeropoulos AP, Georgiopoulou VV, et al. Frailty and risk for heart failure in older adults: the health, aging, and body composition study. Am Heart J 2013;166:887–94.
6. Altimir S, Lupon J, Gonzalez B, et al. Sex and age differences in fragility in a heart failure population. Eur J Heart Fail 2005;7:798–802.
7. Chaudhry SI, McAvay G, Chen S, et al. Risk factors for hospital admission among older persons with newly diagnosed heart failure: findings from the Cardiovascular Health Study. J Am Coll Cardiol 2013; 61:635–42.
8. Dominguez-Rodriguez A, Abreu-Gonzalez P, Jimenez-Sosa A, et al. The impact of frailty in older patients with non-ischaemic cardiomyopathy after implantation of cardiac resynchronization therapy defibrillator. Europace 2015;17:598–602.
9. Dunlay SM, Park SJ, Joyce LD, et al. Frailty and outcomes after implantation of left ventricular assist device as destination therapy. J Heart Lung Transplant 2014;33:359–65.
10. Chung CJ, Wu C, Jones M, et al. Reduced handgrip strength as a marker of frailty predicts clinical outcomes in patients with heart failure undergoing ventricular assist device placement. J Card Fail 2014; 20:310–5.
11. Cruz-Jentoft AJ, Baeyens JP, Bauer JM, et al. Sarcopenia: European consensus on definition and diagnosis: report of the European Working Group on sarcopenia in older people. Age Ageing 2010;39: 412–23.
12. Sullivan MJ, Green HJ, Cobb FR. Skeletal muscle biochemistry and histology in ambulatory patients with long-term heart failure. Circulation 1990;81: 518–27.
13. Evans WJ, Morley JE, Argiles J, et al. Cachexia: a new definition. Clin Nutr 2008;27:793–9.
14. Anker SD, von Haehling S. Inflammatory mediators in chronic heart failure: an overview. Heart 2004; 90:464–70.
15. Walston J, McBurnie MA, Newman A, et al. Frailty and activation of the inflammation and coagulation systems with and without clinical comorbidities: results from the Cardiovascular Health Study. Arch Intern Med 2002;162:2333–41.
16. Phan HM, Alpert JS, Fain M. Frailty, inflammation, and cardiovascular disease: evidence of a connection. Am J Geriatr Cardiol 2008;17:101–7.
17. Anker SD, Ponikowski PP, Clark AL, et al. Cytokines and neurohormones relating to body composition alterations in the wasting syndrome of chronic heart failure. Eur Heart J 1999;20:683–93.
18. Anker SD, Clark AL, Kemp M, et al. Tumor necrosis factor and steroid metabolism in chronic heart failure: possible relation to muscle wasting. J Am Coll Cardiol 1997;30:997–1001.
19. Cicoira M, Kalra PR, Anker SD. Growth hormone resistance in chronic heart failure and its therapeutic implications. J Card Fail 2003;9:219–26.

20. Kalyani RR, Varadhan R, Weiss CO, et al. Frailty status and altered glucose-insulin dynamics. J Gerontol A Biol Sci Med Sci 2012;67:1300–6.

21. Johar H, Emeny RT, Bidlingmaier M, et al. Blunted diurnal cortisol pattern is associated with frailty: a cross-sectional study of 745 participants aged 65 to 90 years. J Clin Endocrinol Metab 2014;99:E464–8.

22. Agapitou V, Dimopoulos S, Kapelios C, et al. Hormonal imbalance in relation to exercise intolerance and ventilatory inefficiency in chronic heart failure. J Heart Lung Transplant 2013;32:431–6.

23. Doehner W, Frenneaux M, Anker SD. Metabolic impairment in heart failure: the myocardial and systemic perspective. J Am Coll Cardiol 2014;64:1388–400.

24. Mohandas A, Reifsnyder J, Jacobs M, et al. Current and future directions in frailty research. Popul Health Manag 2011;14:277–83.

25. Searle SD, Mitnitski A, Gahbauer EA, et al. A standard procedure for creating a frailty index. BMC Geriatr 2008;8:24.

26. Khawaja T, Chokshi A, Ji R, et al. Ventricular assist device implantation improves skeletal muscle function, oxidative capacity, and growth hormone/insulin-like growth factor-1 axis signaling in patients with advanced heart failure. J Cachexia Sarcopenia Muscle 2014;5:297–305.

27. Flint KM, Matlock DD, Lindenfeld J, et al. Frailty and the selection of patients for destination therapy left ventricular assist device. Circ Heart Fail 2012;5:286–93.

28. Lee DH, Buth KJ, Martin BJ, et al. Frail patients are at increased risk for mortality and prolonged institutional care after cardiac surgery. Circulation 2010;121:973–8.

29. Afilalo J, Eisenberg MJ, Morin JF, et al. Gait speed as an incremental predictor of mortality and major morbidity in elderly patients undergoing cardiac surgery. J Am Coll Cardiol 2010;56:1668–76.

30. Lala A, Joyce E, Groarke JD, et al. Challenges in long-term mechanical circulatory support and biological replacement of the failing heart. Circ J 2014;78:288–99.

31. Cowger J, Sundareswaran K, Rogers JG, et al. Predicting survival in patients receiving continuous flow left ventricular assist devices: the HeartMate II risk score. J Am Coll Cardiol 2013;61:313–21.

32. Kirklin JK, Naftel DC, Pagani FD, et al. Seventh INTERMACS annual report: 15,000 patients and counting. J Heart Lung Transplant 2015;34:1495–504.

33. Adamson RM, Stahovich M, Chillcott S, et al. Clinical strategies and outcomes in advanced heart failure patients older than 70 years of age receiving the HeartMate II left ventricular assist device: a community hospital experience. J Am Coll Cardiol 2011;57:2487–95.

34. Lund LH, Edwards LB, Kucheryavaya AY, et al. The Registry of the International Society for Heart and Lung Transplantation: Thirtieth Official Adult Heart Transplant Report–2013; focus theme: age. J Heart Lung Transplant 2013;32:951–64.

35. Cacciatore F, Abete P, Mazzella F, et al. Frailty predicts long-term mortality in elderly subjects with chronic heart failure. Eur J Clin Invest 2005;35:723–30.

36. Leong DP, Teo KK, Rangarajan S, et al. Prognostic value of grip strength: findings from the Prospective Urban Rural Epidemiology (PURE) study. Lancet 2015;386:266–73.

37. Jha SR, Hannu MK, Chang S, et al. The prevalence and prognostic significance of frailty in patients with advanced heart failure referred for heart transplantation. Transplantation 2016;100(2):429–36.

38. Emani S, Brewer RJ, John R, et al. Patients with low compared with high body mass index gain more weight after implantation of a continuous-flow left ventricular assist device. J Heart Lung Transplant 2013;32:31–5.

39. Pulignano G, Del Sindaco D, Di Lenarda A, et al. Usefulness of frailty profile for targeting older heart failure patients in disease management programs: a cost-effectiveness, pilot study. J Cardiovasc Med (Hagerstown) 2010;11:739–47.

40. O'Connor CM, Whellan DJ, Lee KL, et al. Efficacy and safety of exercise training in patients with chronic heart failure: HF-ACTION randomized controlled trial. JAMA 2009;301:1439–50.

41. Flynn KE, Pina IL, Whellan DJ, et al. Effects of exercise training on health status in patients with chronic heart failure: HF-ACTION randomized controlled trial. JAMA 2009;301:1451–9.

42. Cameron ID, Fairhall N, Langron C, et al. A multifactorial interdisciplinary intervention reduces frailty in older people: randomized trial. BMC Med 2013;11:65.

43. Cabilan CJ, Hines S, Munday J. The effectiveness of prehabilitation or preoperative exercise for surgical patients: a systematic review. JBI Database Syst Rev Implement Rep 2015;13:146–87.

44. Rodriguez-Manas L, Feart C, Mann G, et al. Searching for an operational definition of frailty: a Delphi method based consensus statement: the frailty operative definition-consensus conference project. J Gerontol A Biol Sci Med Sci 2013;68:62–7.

45. Rockwood K, Andrew M, Mitnitski A. A comparison of two approaches to measuring frailty in elderly people. J Gerontol A Biol Sci Med Sci 2007;62:738–43.

46. Schmader KE, Hanlon JT, Pieper CF, et al. Effects of geriatric evaluation and management on adverse drug reactions and suboptimal prescribing in the frail elderly. Am J Med 2004;116:394–401.

47. Fiatarone MA, O'Neill EF, Ryan ND, et al. Exercise training and nutritional supplementation for physical

frailty in very elderly people. N Engl J Med 1994;330:1769–75.

48. Latham NK, Bennett DA, Stretton CM, et al. Systematic review of progressive resistance strength training in older adults. J Gerontol A Biol Sci Med Sci 2004;59:48–61.

49. Scherer M, Dungen HD, Inkrot S, et al. Determinants of change in quality of life in the Cardiac Insufficiency Bisoprolol Study in Elderly (CIBIS-ELD). Eur J Intern Med 2013;24:333–8.

50. Toma M, McAlister FA, Coglianese EE, et al. Testosterone supplementation in heart failure: a meta-analysis. Circ Heart Fail 2012;5:315–21.

51. Morley JE, Vellas B, van Kan GA, et al. Frailty consensus: a call to action. J Am Med Dir Assoc 2013;14:392–7.

Tailoring Therapies in Advanced Heart Failure

Carrie Puckett, DO, James O. Mudd, MD*

KEYWORDS

• Advanced heart failure • Hemodynamics • Tailored therapy • Pulmonary artery catheter

KEY POINTS

- Define advanced heart failure.
- Discuss tailoring medical therapies and monitoring of patients with advanced heart failure.
- Discuss decision making and goals of care discussions in advanced heart failure and how these conversations guide therapies.

Heart failure (HF) is a growing epidemic affecting millions of people and significantly impacts the economics and systems of care delivery and will only become more complex with an aging population.[1] Various etiologies lead to this clinical syndrome, which is progressive and characterized by labile degrees of severity. As medical and device therapies have extended life with HF, there are increasing proportions of patients surviving to have advanced HF. Advanced HF is defined as chronic HF that has progressed to symptoms with minimal exertion or at rest (New York Heart Association [NYHA] class III or class IV) with periods of decompensation despite optimized medical, device, and surgical therapies.[2] Functional impairment can be defined as a 6-minute walk test less than or equal to 300 m or peak oxygen consumption less than 12 mL/kg/min to 14 mL/kg/min.[3] When defining advanced HF, life expectancy with HF should also be considered and can be approximated using risk models, such as the Seattle HF Model or the Heart Failure Survival Score.[4] Important clinical features of advanced HF include recurrent HF hospitalizations, unintentional weight loss, declining renal function, intolerance to neurohormonal antagonists, escalating diuretic doses, hypotension, and hyponatremia.[3] Such milestones should prompt consideration of referral to a HF program with access to advanced therapies.

The goal of therapy in advanced HF is to improve quality of life and prolong survival. Invasive hemodynamic assessment has been a cornerstone in defining and measuring hemodynamic responses to therapeutic interventions to augment cardiac output, reduce systemic vascular resistance, and improve neurohormonal activation, resulting in better functional status and quality of life in patients with advanced HF.[5,6] As the disease progresses, many standard medical therapies may require tailoring as advanced therapies, such as transplant and mechanical circulatory support, are considered in the context of patient and caregiver goals. The pathway to improved quality and quantity of life for the growing population of patients with advanced HF is highly variable, and careful tailoring of medical, psychosocial, and systems interventions is critical. The aim of this review is to summarize concepts for tailored medical therapy and monitoring in advanced HF and discuss the importance of tailoring systems of care and shared decision making in advanced HF.

Knight Cardiovascular Institute, Oregon Health and Science University, 3181 Southwest Sam Jackson Park Road, UHN 62, Portland, OR 97239, USA
* Correspondence author. Knight Cardiovascular Institute, Oregon Health and Science University, 3181 Southwest Sam Jackson Park Road, UHN 62, Portland, OR 97239.
E-mail address: mudd@ohsu.edu

Heart Failure Clin 12 (2016) 375–384
http://dx.doi.org/10.1016/j.hfc.2016.03.009
1551-7136/16/$ – see front matter © 2016 Elsevier Inc. All rights reserved.

OPTIMIZING MEDICAL THERAPY IN ADVANCED HF

One of the cornerstones of chronic HF management is to improve congestive symptoms with diuretics and hemodynamic conditions so as to maximize perfusion with vasodilators (eg, neurohormonal antagonists). This requires constant surveillance and re-evaluation for exacerbating factors, which are common in patients with advanced HF. Although randomized clinical trials have demonstrated improved survival and quality of life in HF, many patients with advanced HF seen in ambulatory practice or hospitalized with acute exacerbations reside outside clinical trial enrollment criteria.[7] A majority of randomized HF studies have primarily enrolled NYHA II–III patients, although there have been several studies focused on NYHA III–IV patients (Table 1). Despite the severity of their condition, as the disease progresses, these patients derive benefit from optimizing medical therapy with careful attention to dosing and the balance of medication classes.

Angiotensin-converting enzyme inhibitors (ACEIs) are first-line agents in patients with HF and reduced ejection fraction, independent of clinical symptoms. Numerous large randomized trials have demonstrated improved activity tolerance and symptoms, with reductions in mortality and cardiovascular hospitalizations.[8,9] Treatment should be initiated at low doses with further titration based on symptoms, blood pressure, and renal function. The use of short-acting captopril can be maximized in an acute decompensated state where tolerance and rapid titration can be monitored. The titration of ACEI therapy may be limited by blood pressure but should be titrated to the highest tolerated dose because higher doses are associated with less hospitalization.[10] These agents remain recommended in individuals with chronic kidney disease as long as the estimated glomerular filtration rate is greater than 30 mL/min/1.73 m^2.[3] In the landmark Cooperative North Scandinavian Enalapril Survival Study (CONSENSUS) trial of enalapril in NYHA IV patients, there was a 31% relative risk reduction in mortality at 1 year and a 50% reduction in progressive HF death. Angiotensin II receptor blockers (ARBs) have also been shown to improve symptoms and mortality and reduce hospitalizations in NYHA II–IV HF patients[11,12] and can be used as an alternative to ACEIs, although lack of short-acting formulations can limit their use when relative hypotension is present. In the advanced stages of HF, there may be concerns for renal insufficiency, hypotension, or hyperkalemia that preclude the use of ACEI/ARB therapy. Patients who fall into this category have a greater than 50% one year, thus identifying a subset of patients with particularly severe and advanced HF.[13]

For patients who are intolerant to ACEI/ARB or who have enough blood pressure to support further vasodilation, hydralazine and isosorbide dinitrate (ISDN) can be effective vasodilators to further improve preload and afterload conditions. Initially studied in the landmark Vasodilator–Heart Failure Trial (V-HeFT), hydralazine and nitrates were shown to be beneficial in improving exercise capacity and survival.[14] A signal of benefit in African American patients in V-HeFT I and V-HeFT II led to a trial focused on this population.[15] The African-American Heart Failure Trial (A-HeFT) study randomized self-identified African American individuals with NYHA III–IV HF already receiving background medical therapy with ACEI/ARB, β-blockers, aldosterone blocker, digoxin, and diuretics to a combination pill of hydralazine and ISDN.[16] This trial was stopped prematurely due to a significant 43% relative reduction in mortality in this advanced HF population.[16] In clinical practice, hydralazine and nitrates are often used in patients presenting with acute HF syndromes who have relative contraindications to continuing or starting ACEI/ARB therapies yet would benefit from initiation of oral vasodilators. Adjunctive

Table 1
Heart failure medical trials enrolling New York Heart Association class III–IV patients

Trial	New York Heart Association Class	Drug	Mortality Relative Risk Reduction (%)
CONSENSUS I	NYHA–IV	Enalapril vs placebo	31
CIBIS II	NYHA III–IV	Bisoprolol vs placebo	34
COPERNICUS	NYHA–IV	Carvedilol vs placebo	35
RALES	NYHA III–IV	Spironolactone vs placebo	30
A-HeFT	NYHA III–IV	ISDN + hydralazine vs placebo	43

Abbreviation: CIBIS, cardiac insufficiency bisoprolol study.

medical therapy for advanced HF also includes digoxin, which can decrease hospitalizations without a significant change in mortality, although they have not been studied in acute decompensated advanced HF.[17]

In addition to ACEIs, β-blockers are key treatments to further modifying the enhanced adrenergic and neurohormonal signals in chronic HF. Across the spectrum of NYHA II–IV HF, β-blockers decrease HF symptom burden and reduce the risk of death and HF hospitalization.[18–21] Their role in advanced HF is more nuanced. The Carvedilol Prospective Randomized Cumulative Survival (COPERNICUS) study focused on euvolemic NYHA III–IV patients and demonstrated a significant reduction in mortality and HF hospitalization as well as fewer days hospitalized.[18,22] Patients also had improved symptom burden and decreased adverse events, such as worsening HF, cardiogenic shock, or sudden death.[18] β-Blockers should be used cautiously, however, in advanced HF and may not be tolerated. For example, in the medical arm of the Randomized Evaluation of Mechanical Assistance for the Treatment of Congestive Heart Failure (REMATCH) trial of destination left ventricular assist device (LVAD) versus medical therapy, fewer than 30% of patients in the medical arm were on β-blockers, likely due to intolerance reflected by the high use of inotropic support.[23]

The 3 agents shown effective in reducing mortality in HF patients in randomized trials are bisoprolol, metoprolol succinate, and carvedilol. In advanced HF, blood pressure may limit the use of these agents; dosing different agents at different times of day to try to maintain β-blocker therapy should be considered. β-Blocker withdrawal is associated with worse outcomes during HF hospitalizations but this observation is likely a marker of disease severity rather than a driver of the worse outcomes.[24] As with ACEI, β-blockers should be initiated at low doses and in the absence of significant volume overload and slowly titrated for patients with recent decompensation. Patients should be well compensated prior to initiation of β-blockers; yet every attempt should be made to ensure patients are on β-blockers prior to discharge because this leads to improved postdischarge mortality.[24] It should be recognized, however, that some advanced HF patients may not tolerate even the lowest doses of β-blockade due to excessive hypotension, persistent congestion, or unrecognized low-output states.

Long-term therapy with aldosterone receptor antagonists has been shown to reduce morbidity and mortality along the entire spectrum of HF severity classes, including advanced HF.[25,26] The Randomized Aldactone Evaluation Study (RALES) trial studied NYHA III–IV patients on ACEI/ARBs and β-blockers to assess further neurohormonal inhibition with spironolactone. Patients randomized to spironolactone had a 30% reduction in all-cause mortality and 35% reduction in hospitalizations for worsening HF.[25] Renal function and potassium levels at baseline must be considered prior to initiation and closely monitored thereafter, which are particularly critical clinical practice issues in the advanced HF patient.[3] Aldosterone receptor antagonist doses may be increased in advanced HF patients who have high diuretic and potassium needs to doses not studied in the clinical trials, but the safety and efficacy of this approach are unproved.

Loop diuretics are a cornerstone of HF management, regardless of the severity of HF. There are particular nuances of diuretic management, however, in advanced HF that are worth noting. The most commonly used oral loop diuretic is furosemide; yet, this diuretic is bound to albumin, which is often reduced in patients with advanced HF. Advanced HF is almost always associated with cardiorenal syndrome and the renal braking phenomenon; it is clinically important that adequate doses of diuretics are used. Patients with advanced HF also have altered gut absorptive function and, therefore, decreased oral bioavailability of certain drugs; torsemide or bumetanide may be better than furosemide in this regard and provide longer and more predictable duration of action. Thiazide diuretics may be beneficial for sequential nephron blockade when used before a loop diuretic to block distal tubular reabsorption of sodium. Increasing doses of diuretics or the need for routine thiazide diuretics to relieve congestion is a sign of advancing HF and is associated with increased mortality.

INVASIVE HEMODYNAMIC TAILORED THERAPY

Throughout the progression of HF, a constant reassessment of volume and functional status is critical. Some patients are labeled as intolerant to a medication but it may be due to an inaccurate bedside assessment of volume status and cardiac output and not necessarily the drug itself. Such scenarios should prompt clinicians to consider invasive hemodynamic assessment. Pulmonary artery catheterization (PAC) provides the definitive hemodynamic picture when there is diagnostic uncertainty and can also be used to continuously to guide therapy (**Box 1**).[27] Although commonly considered during a HF hospitalization, clinicians

---

Box 1
Indications for pulmonary artery catheter use in advanced HF

Acute cardiogenic shock requiring vasoactive agents or temporary mechanical support

Inability to accurately assess hemodynamics with impaired perfusion

Unclear hemodynamic state despite attempts at medical optimization

Persistent symptoms despite attempts at medical optimization

Suspected right-sided HF > left-sided HF

Reassess hemodynamics after inotropic support to improve clinical status

Evaluation for heart transplant or long-term mechanical support

---

should consider such an approach for ambulatory patients when tailored therapy may allow greater dose titration of commonly used HF therapies.

Invasive hemodynamic monitoring can play a key role in the management of advanced HF. The PAC has a storied history in cardiovascular medicine and was adopted for its ease of use in critical care settings.[28] With widespread use, however, came increased scrutiny and the eventual call for randomized trials to demonstrate benefit. Perhaps surprisingly, such trials have yet to demonstrate benefit with increased complications in critically ill medical and surgical patients.[29,30] To better define the role of the PAC in patients hospitalized with acute decompensated HF, the Evaluation Study of Congestive Heart Failure and Pulmonary Artery Catheterization Effectiveness (ESCAPE) study was conducted. The goal of the study was to enroll patients with advanced HF who were thought ill enough such that PAC was appropriate but stable enough to continue care without one, for example, clinical equipoise.[31] Use of inotropic support was discouraged and patients who were thought to need PAC for urgent management were excluded from the study. The trial randomized 433 patients to usual care with PAC compared with usual care alone. There was no difference in the primary endpoint of the number of days alive outside the hospital at 6 months, with more in-hospital adverse events in the PAC group.[32]

In ESCAPE, however, there were specific subgroups that were of note. For example, use of PAC to guide therapy with the intravenous vasodilator sodium nitroprusside in patients with advanced HF and low cardiac index (<2.0 L/min/m^2) resulted in higher doses of oral vasodilators,

greater reductions in central filling pressures without more use of inotropes, or worsening renal function.[33] Patients treated with sodium nitroprusside had lower all-cause mortality and no increase in rehospitalization rates.[33] Therefore, although the ESCAPE trial did not demonstrate a benefit for routine PAC-guided therapy for acute decompensated HF, the PAC can still help guide clinicians in carefully selected advanced HF patients. Such patients include those who are not responding to routine therapies or who have progressive symptoms despite optimal medical therapy.[3,32,34]

Once invasively defined, the hemodynamic picture may help guide further management strategies. In the ESCAPE trial, clinicians were good at assessing right-sided and left-sided filling pressures as well as a general sense of the cardiac output based on a cold or warm profile, yet even the warm profile had a low resting cardiac index of 2.0 L/min/m^2.[34] In this example, the invasively assessed hemodynamic profile might suggest a need for augmentation of cardiac output with oral or intravenous vasodilators that might not have been appreciated at the bedside. Moreover, unrecognized or underappreciated congestion may be discovered and further diuresis may be warranted. Finally, quantifying the severity of pulmonary hypertension that bears impact on oral therapies as well as an impact on the suitability for advanced therapies, such as transplant or mechanical support, is always critical information that may not have been apparent from a noninvasive evaluation.[3]

PAC-guided management is directed toward specific hemodynamic goals that should translate into symptomatic benefit (as discussed previously) in the ESCAPE trial. When this approach is taken, active management of the PAC-acquired data is critical to continually assess response to therapies and to justify the risks of an indwelling vascular catheter. In general, diuretics and vasodilators are used to lower filling pressures (eg, central venous pressure [CVP] <8 mm Hg and pulmonary capillary wedge [PCW] <16 mm Hg) and resistance to specific targets (**Table 2**). Patients who present with elevated filling pressures, an elevated systemic vascular resistance (eg, >1800–2000 dyne/s/cm^5) and a concomitantly low cardiac index may benefit in a dramatic fashion from a balanced intravenous vasodilator, such as sodium nitroprusside, as a bridge to oral vasodilators. At times, inotropic support is necessary for combinations of low cardiac index and minimal elevations in systemic vascular resistance, with the same goal of transitioning to oral therapies while maintaining adequate filling pressures and mean arterial pressure. Choice of inotropic support may

Table 2	
Suggested hemodynamic goals in advanced HF	
Goal	**Hemodynamic Parameter**
Maintain blood pressure	SBP $\geq$80–90 mm Hg, MAP $\geq$65 mm Hg
Decrease right-sided filling pressures	CVP <8 mm Hg
Decrease left-sided filling pressures	PCW <16 mm Hg
Decrease peripheral resistance	SVR 1000–1200 dyne/s/cm^{-5}
Decrease pulmonary resistance	Mean PA $\geq$25% reduction, PVR <3 WU, TPG <15 mm Hg
Increase cardiac output	Cardiac index $\geq$2.2 L/min/m^2

Abbreviations: MAP, mean arterial pressure; PA, pulmonary artery; PVR, pulmonary vascular resistance; SBP, systolic blood pressure; SVR, systemic vascular resistance; TPG, transpulmonary gradient; WU, wood units.

depend on several factors, including blood pressure, arrhythmias, and renal function. Although there are no studies supporting the routine and long-term use of intropic support in HF, this therapy can help alleviated symptoms, improve hemodynamics, and bridge patients to further treatment options, such as LVAD or transplant. When patients are unable to be weaned from intravenous therapies without hemodynamic compromise and deemed inotropic dependent, however, they have poor short-term outcomes.[35] Further use of inotropic support in advanced HF is discussed elsewhere in this issue (see Ginwalla M: Home Inotropes and Other Palliative Care, in this issue). Proposed invasive hemodynamic goals in advanced HF are listed in **Table 2**.

Invasive hemodynamic assessment is also critical for advanced HF patients who are candidates for mechanical support. For example, equalized filling pressures of the right atrium and PCW are risk factors for acute and chronic right ventricular (RV) dysfunction after LVAD placement.[36] Other hemodynamic parameters have been derived to assess risk for early RV mechanical support after LVAD implant, including RV stroke work index, tricuspid annular plane systolic excursion, and pulmonary artery pulsatility index.[37,38]

An invasive hemodynamic snapshot may also be useful for the so-called walking wounded (ie, Interagency Registry for Mechanically Assisted Circulatory Support [INTERMACS] profile 6) advanced HF patients who somehow avoid hospitalization but have a high symptom burden with frequent medication modifications and labile renal function.

In these situations, an invasive assessment may help tailor the pathway beyond medical therapy, such as consideration for heart transplant, mechanical support, or hospice in patients deemed optimally treated.

IMPLANTABLE AMBULATORY HEMODYNAMIC MONITORING

Although the PAC plays an important role in evaluating patients with end-stage HF, it has some practical limitations, such as the need for hospitalization. Over the past decade, numerous devices have been developed to provide surrogate or direct measures of left atrial and pulmonary pressures for ambulatory monitoring. These devices have been predominately studied in less sick, chronic HF patients, and data are lacking in a true advanced HF cohort. The first such device for remote hemodynamic monitoring was based on using RV leads for cardiac resynchronization therapy or implantable cardioverter-defibrillator devices and used algorithms to provide estimated pulmonary artery diastolic pressure or thoracic impedance as metrics of central congestion. Use of the Chronicle device (Medtronic, St. Paul, MN) in a randomized, single-blind controlled trial in NYHA III–IV patients led to a nonsignificant trend in reducing HF related events, including HF hospitalizations.[39] Despite the nonsignificant results of the primary endpoint and ultimate lack of Food and Drug Association approval in the United States, this study was an important contribution to the use of hemodynamic monitoring in ambulatory patients to optimize HF therapy. Other devices have followed. For example, a left atrial pressure (LAP) monitor in NYHA III–IV patients helped tailor therapy to lower LAP with subsequent improvements in NYHA class and ejection fraction.[40]

With advances in sensor technology, smaller, fully implantable, nontethered devices are now available for remote hemodynamic monitoring. The CardioMEMS (St. Jude Medical, St. Paul, MN) sensor is a wireless, leadless sensor without a battery implanted into the pulmonary artery. The patient rests on an external antenna, which powers the device and transforms the frequency data into a pressure waveform. The device was studied in

550 patients with NYHA III HF and a prior HF admission (regardless of ejection fraction) in a randomized fashion to usual care plus pulmonary artery sensor data to usual care alone.[41] As with all pieces of discrete data, the process and algorithm to act on the data were a critical and important part of this study. Compared with standard of care, patients with the CardioMEMS device had a 39% reduction in HF hospitalizations over an average follow-up of 15 months.[41] For patients who have advanced HF, these devices may provide additional information outside of the clinic that can be used to tailor therapies to specific hemodynamic goals to decrease symptom burden and HF–related hospitalizations.

TAILORING PATHWAYS TO LEFT VENTRICULAR ASSIST DEVICE/TRANSPLANT

In the current era, the prospects for transplant have changed. As heart transplant wait lists grow, so have wait list times in the United States; however, wait list mortality has improved, largely due to the improved survival that current continuous flow LVADs provide.[42] Thus, tailoring the pathway to transplant/LVAD depends on many variables that have an impact on post-transplant outcomes and wait list mortality.[43] For example, not all patients are good candidates for LVAD, such as those with restrictive/hypertrophic cardiomyopathies, where small left ventricular dimensions and mild reductions in ejection fraction result in small stroke volumes and often difficult-to-reduce filling pressures. Similarly, patients with adult congenital heart disease are poor candidates for mechanical circulatory support due to multiple prior sternotomies, pulmonary hypertension, and protein-losing enteropathies and often wait as inpatients for prolonged periods of time for transplant.[44] Other patients with advanced HF may be poor candidates for transplant or LVAD due to other medical or psychosocial contraindications. As such, there is a current proposal to modify the current heart allocation system to better reflect patient subsets who are not candidates for mechanical assist but are no less ill (see Kittleson: Changing Role of Heart Transplantation, in this issue).[45,46] Providers should communicate that the improved survival with these therapies come with requisite increased short-term and long-term risks and that these considerations have to be tailored to patients, their caretakers, and their goals.

TAILORING TO QUALITY OF LIFE

Gaps still exist in the understanding of patient preferences and the use of nonpharmacologic interventions to improve HF outcomes. A key to managing chronic and advanced HF is understanding and managing patient expectations. Compared with predicted life expectancy modeling with the Seattle Heart Failure Model, patients with NYHA III–IV HF overestimate their life expectancy by up to 3 years.[47] Similarly, understanding whether a patient would trade time for quality has a modest relationship to symptom burden and most patients favor survival, which only improves after HF discharge.[48] Metrics of frailty, adherence, and access to care are only a few of many factors that have an impact on patient engagement and the ability to manage complex medical and lifestyle regimens. Little investigation has been done in patient-tailored education beyond the requisite salt and fluid restriction goals that ironically lack a strong evidence base (although they are in line with pathophysiologic understanding of the disease). New avenues for structured patient education and counseling may improve HF outcomes throughout the spectrum of the disease and should be a focus of tailoring treatments in patients with advanced HF.[49] Discussing advanced therapies, such as destination LVAD, with patients and caregivers is a daunting and intimidating task, yet setting expectations is critical for patient engagement and decision making. This process is often fragmented with no defined standards and commonly lacks feedback. To better understand this process, the DECIDE-LVAD (Trial of a Decision Support Intervention for Patients and Caregivers Offered Destination Therapy Heart Assist Device) study is being performed to assess a scripted education process to improve patient and caregiver experiences and decision quality (https://clinicaltrials.gov/ct2/show/NCT02344576).

TAILORING THE TEAM TO THE PATIENT

Beyond evidence-based pharmacologic and device therapies, a cornerstone to HF management remains the constituents of the team and the dyadic relationship between the patient and team to monitor the disease course and consider treatment options (**Fig. 1**). In general, patients undergoing formal transplant/LVAD evaluation have much more rigorous monitoring than patients less ill who are not currently candidates for transplant or LVAD. But what of patients who are not transplant candidates or not recognized to need a transplant/LVAD evaluation? These individuals are no less ill and their care needs tailoring not only in terms of HF clinic visits but also the constituents and resources for those visits.[50] A key aspect of tailoring therapy for any stage of HF is the nature

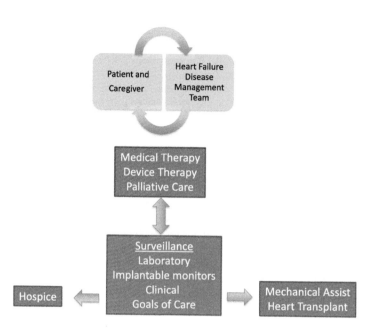

Fig. 1. Dyadic relationship between patient and HF team to engage in shared decision making and monitoring to inform advanced therapy options.

of the team and their plan to have these individual aspects reviewed at routine intervals in a layered fashion to achieve patient directed goals.[51] As the disease progresses and considerations for LVAD, transplant, or hospice come to the forefront, careful decisions and counseling within the team and with the patient are needed, given the inherent risks of these therapies.[47] Thus, a tailored decision-making process is necessary not only for the patient and care providers but also for the team itself so a patient's quality of life and choices are openly understood and followed.[52,53] This approach requires a comprehensive disease management team skilled not only in cardiovascular medicine but also in nutrition, exercise science, palliative care, psychology, and social work, with meticulous care coordination to respond to patients dynamic needs.

TAILORING EXPECTATIONS

Patients with advanced HF can be inundated with complex medication schedules, dietary restrictions, device-monitoring algorithms, exercise prescriptions, and frequent clinical and laboratory visits, which themselves are tailored to the heterogeneity of the disease. Sometimes lost in the prescriptions for monitoring and treatments are the crucial conversations about the goals of the therapies and how they best align with patient goals and the balance of quality versus quantity of life. Given the progressive unpredictable nature of the disease, it is important to have these conversations

in earlier stages of HF so expectations are clear and goals are continually addressed in a systematic manner.[47] This ensures an open and evolving dialogue as to patient and family preferences based on external life events and new therapies and through the obligate periods of calm punctuated by periods of unrest that are the hallmark of advanced HF.

As medical therapies have improved mortality in HF, a growing population of patients is surviving into the advanced stages of the condition with complex comorbid conditions and considerations. Identification of key clinical variables signaling a transition to advanced HF can trigger early referral to comprehensive HF teams to discuss the options for relieving symptoms, improving quality of life, and extending longevity. Therapies that were once tolerable may become intolerable and constant reevaluation is necessary. Not all patients are candidates for heart transplant or LVADs and understanding patient goals of care is critical in tailoring a treatment plan. The paucity of data in well-constructed clinical trials of medical therapy in advanced HF results in a greater need to individualize therapeutic approaches based on patient/caretaker goals, provider experience, and local resources and culture.

REFERENCES

1. Heidenreich PA, Albert NM, Allen LA, et al. Forecasting the impact of heart failure in the United States: a policy statement from the

American Heart Association. Circ Heart Fail 2013; 6(3):606–19.

2. Fang JC, Ewald GA, Allen LA, et al. Advanced (stage D) heart failure: a statement from the Heart Failure Society of America Guidelines Committee. J Card Fail 2015;21(6):519–34.

3. Writing Committee Members, Yancy CW, Jessup M, Bozkurt B, et al. 2013 ACCF/AHA guideline for the management of heart failure: a report of the American College of Cardiology Foundation/American Heart Association Task Force on practice guidelines. Circulation 2013;128(16):e240–327.

4. Levy WC, Mozaffarian D, Linker DT, et al. The Seattle Heart Failure Model: prediction of survival in heart failure. Circulation 2006;113(11):1424–33.

5. Stevenson LW, Tillisch JH, Hamilton M, et al. Importance of hemodynamic response to therapy in predicting survival with ejection fraction less than or equal to 20% secondary to ischemic or nonischemic dilated cardiomyopathy. Am J Cardiol 1990;66(19):1348–54.

6. Stevenson LW, Tillisch JH. Maintenance of cardiac output with normal filling pressures in patients with dilated heart failure. Circulation 1986;74(6):1303–8.

7. Masoudi FA, Havranek EP, Wolfe P, et al. Most hospitalized older persons do not meet the enrollment criteria for clinical trials in heart failure. Am Heart J 2003;146(2):250–7.

8. Effects of enalapril on mortality in severe congestive heart failure. Results of the Cooperative North Scandinavian Enalapril Survival Study (CONSENSUS). The CONSENSUS Trial Study Group. N Engl J Med 1987;316(23):1429–35.

9. Effect of enalapril on survival in patients with reduced left ventricular ejection fractions and congestive heart failure. The SOLVD Investigators. N Engl J Med 1991;325(5):293–302.

10. Packer M, Poole-Wilson PA, Armstrong PW, et al. Comparative effects of low and high doses of the angiotensin-converting enzyme inhibitor, lisinopril, on morbidity and mortality in chronic heart failure. ATLAS Study Group. Circulation 1999;100(23):2312–8.

11. Granger CB, McMurray JJ, Yusuf S, et al. Effects of candesartan in patients with chronic heart failure and reduced left-ventricular systolic function intolerant to angiotensin-converting-enzyme inhibitors: the CHARM-Alternative trial. Lancet 2003; 362(9386):772–6.

12. Cohn JN, Tognoni G, Valsartan Heart Failure Trial Investigators. A randomized trial of the angiotensin-receptor blocker valsartan in chronic heart failure. N Engl J Med 2001;345(23):1667–75.

13. Kittleson M, Hurwitz S, Shah MR, et al. Development of circulatory-renal limitations to angiotensin-converting enzyme inhibitors identifies patients with severe heart failure and early mortality. J Am Coll Cardiol 2003;41(11):2029–35.

14. Cohn JN, Archibald DG, Ziesche S, et al. Effect of vasodilator therapy on mortality in chronic congestive heart failure. Results of a Veterans Administration Cooperative Study. N Engl J Med 1986;314(24):1547–52.

15. Carson P, Ziesche S, Johnson G, et al. Racial differences in response to therapy for heart failure: analysis of the vasodilator-heart failure trials. Vasodilator-Heart Failure Trial Study Group. J Card Fail 1999;5(3):178–87.

16. Taylor AL, Ziesche S, Yancy C, et al. Combination of isosorbide dinitrate and hydralazine in blacks with heart failure. N Engl J Med 2004;351(20):2049–57.

17. The Digitalis Investigation Group. The effect of digoxin on mortality and morbidity in patients with heart failure. N Engl J Med 1997;336(8):525–33.

18. Packer M, Fowler MB, Roecker EB, et al. Effect of carvedilol on the morbidity of patients with severe chronic heart failure: results of the carvedilol prospective randomized cumulative survival (COPERNICUS) study. Circulation 2002;106(17):2194–9.

19. Poole-Wilson PA, Swedberg K, Cleland JG, et al. Comparison of carvedilol and metoprolol on clinical outcomes in patients with chronic heart failure in the Carvedilol Or Metoprolol European Trial (COMET): randomised controlled trial. Lancet 2003;362(9377):7–13.

20. The Cardiac Insufficiency Bisoprolol Study II (CIBIS-II): a randomised trial. Lancet 1999;353(9146):9–13.

21. Effect of metoprolol CR/XL in chronic heart failure: Metoprolol CR/XL Randomised Intervention Trial in Congestive Heart Failure (MERIT-HF). Lancet 1999; 353(9169):2001–7.

22. Packer M, Coats AJ, Fowler MB, et al. Effect of carvedilol on survival in severe chronic heart failure. N Engl J Med 2001;344(22):1651–8.

23. Rose EA, Gelijns AC, Moskowitz AJ, et al. Long-term use of a left ventricular assist device for end-stage heart failure. N Engl J Med 2001;345(20):1435–43.

24. Fonarow GC, Abraham WT, Albert NM, et al. Influence of beta-blocker continuation or withdrawal on outcomes in patients hospitalized with heart failure: findings from the OPTIMIZE-HF program. J Am Coll Cardiol 2008;52(3):190–9.

25. Pitt B, Zannad F, Remme WJ, et al. The effect of spironolactone on morbidity and mortality in patients with severe heart failure. Randomized Aldactone Evaluation Study Investigators. N Engl J Med 1999;341(10):709–17.

26. Zannad F, McMurray JJ, Krum H, et al. Eplerenone in patients with systolic heart failure and mild symptoms. N Engl J Med 2011;364(1):11–21.

27. Nohria A, Tsang SW, Fang JC, et al. Clinical assessment identifies hemodynamic profiles that predict outcomes in patients admitted with heart failure. J Am Coll Cardiol 2003;41(10):1797–804.

28. Chatterjee K. The Swan-Ganz catheters: past, present, and future. A viewpoint. Circulation 2009; 119(1):147–52.

29. Sandham JD, Hull RD, Brant RF, et al. A randomized, controlled trial of the use of pulmonary-artery catheters in high-risk surgical patients. N Engl J Med 2003;348(1):5–14.

30. Harvey S, Harrison DA, Singer M, et al. Assessment of the clinical effectiveness of pulmonary artery catheters in management of patients in intensive care (PAC-Man): a randomised controlled trial. Lancet 2005;366(9484):472–7.

31. Shah MR, O'Connor CM, Sopko G, et al. Evaluation Study of Congestive Heart Failure and Pulmonary Artery Catheterization Effectiveness (ESCAPE): design and rationale. Am Heart J 2001;141(4): 528–35.

32. Binanay C, Califf RM, Hasselblad V, et al. Evaluation study of congestive heart failure and pulmonary artery catheterization effectiveness: the ESCAPE trial. JAMA 2005;294(13):1625–33.

33. Mullens W, Abrahams Z, Francis GS, et al. Sodium nitroprusside for advanced low-output heart failure. J Am Coll Cardiol 2008;52(3):200–7.

34. Drazner MH, Hellkamp AS, Leier CV, et al. Value of clinician assessment of hemodynamics in advanced heart failure: the ESCAPE trial. Circ Heart Fail 2008; 1(3):170–7.

35. Hershberger RE, Nauman D, Walker TL, et al. Care processes and clinical outcomes of continuous outpatient support with inotropes (COSI) in patients with refractory endstage heart failure. J Card Fail 2003;9(3):180–7.

36. Matthews JC, Koelling TM, Pagani FD, et al. The right ventricular failure risk score a pre-operative tool for assessing the risk of right ventricular failure in left ventricular assist device candidates. J Am Coll Cardiol 2008;51(22): 2163–72.

37. Kormos RL, Teuteberg JJ, Pagani FD, et al. Right ventricular failure in patients with the Heart-Mate II continuous-flow left ventricular assist device: incidence, risk factors, and effect on outcomes. J Thorac Cardiovasc Surg 2010; 139(5):1316–24.

38. Kang G, Ha R, Banerjee D. Pulmonary artery pulsatility index predicts right ventricular failure after left ventricular assist device implantation. J Heart Lung Transplant 2016;35(1):67–73.

39. Bourge RC, Abraham WT, Adamson PB, et al. Randomized controlled trial of an implantable continuous hemodynamic monitor in patients with advanced heart failure: the COMPASS-HF study. J Am Coll Cardiol 2008;51(11):1073–9.

40. Ritzema J, Melton IC, Richards AM, et al. Direct left atrial pressure monitoring in ambulatory heart failure patients: initial experience with a new permanent implantable device. Circulation 2007;116(25): 2952–9.

41. Adamson PB, Abraham WT, Aaron M, et al. CHAMPION trial rationale and design: the long-term safety and clinical efficacy of a wireless pulmonary artery pressure monitoring system. J Card Fail 2011;17(1):3–10.

42. Schulze PC, Kitada S, Clerkin K, et al. Regional differences in recipient waitlist time and pre- and posttransplant mortality after the 2006 United Network for Organ Sharing policy changes in the donor heart allocation algorithm. JACC Heart Fail 2014; 2(2):166–77.

43. Singh TP, Milliren CE, Almond CS, et al. Survival benefit from transplantation in patients listed for heart transplantation in the United States. J Am Coll Cardiol 2014;63(12):1169–78.

44. Gelow JM, Song HK, Weiss JB, et al. Organ allocation in adults with congenital heart disease listed for heart transplant: impact of ventricular assist devices. J Heart Lung Transplant 2013;32(11): 1059–64.

45. Kobashigawa JA, Johnson M, Rogers J, et al. Report from a forum on US heart allocation policy. Am J Transplant 2015;15(1):55–63.

46. Meyer DM, Rogers JG, Edwards LB, et al. The future direction of the adult heart allocation system in the United States. Am J Transplant 2015; 15(1):44–54.

47. Allen LA, Stevenson LW, Grady KL, et al. Decision making in advanced heart failure: a scientific statement from the American Heart Association. Circulation 2012;125(15):1928–52.

48. Stevenson LW, Hellkamp AS, Leier CV, et al. Changing preferences for survival after hospitalization with advanced heart failure. J Am Coll Cardiol 2008; 52(21):1702–8.

49. Masterson Creber R, Patey M, Lee CS, et al. Motivational interviewing to improve self-care for patients with chronic heart failure: MITI-HF randomized controlled trial. Patient Educ Couns 2016;99(2): 256–64.

50. Wever-Pinzon O, Drakos SG, Fang JC. Team-based care for advanced heart failure. Heart Fail Clin 2015; 11(3):467–77.

51. Grady KL, Dracup K, Kennedy G, et al. Team management of patients with heart failure: a statement for healthcare professionals from The Cardiovascular Nursing Council of the American Heart Association. Circulation 2000; 102(19):2443–56.

52. McIlvennan CK, Jones J, Allen LA, et al. Decision-making for destination therapy left ventricular assist devices: implications for caregivers. Circ Cardiovasc Qual Outcomes 2015;8(2):172–8.

53. Stewart GC, Brooks K, Pratibhu PP, et al. Thresholds of physical activity and life expectancy for patients considering destination ventricular assist devices. J Heart Lung Transplant 2009;28(9):863–9.

Temporary Percutaneous Mechanical Circulatory Support in Advanced Heart Failure

Jessica L. Brown, MD[a], Jerry D. Estep, MD[b],*

KEYWORDS

- Cardiogenic shock • Percutaneous mechanical circulatory support • IABP • Impella • TandemHeart
- ECMO • Pressure-volume loop

KEY POINTS

- Temporary percutaneous mechanical circulatory support (MCS) devices are increasingly used for patients with cardiogenic shock as a bridge to recovery, decision, or definitive therapy.
- Temporary percutaneous MCS devices include the intra-aortic balloon pump, TandemHeart, Impella, and extracorporeal membrane oxygenation.
- The choice of MCS device is multifactorial, based on patient characteristics, operator ability, and the degree of hemodynamic support desired.
- The hemodynamic effects vary across the MCS device types and are an important consideration when evaluating a patient's response to MCS support.
- The use of temporary MCS is best approached through a care team that includes an advanced heart failure cardiologist.

Temporary percutaneous mechanical circulatory support (MCS) is part of the treatment armamentarium for high-risk percutaneous intervention (PCI) and acute myocardial infarction (AMI) complicated with cardiogenic shock.[1] Cardiogenic shock is typically defined as severe, refractory heart failure caused by significant myocardial dysfunction in the setting of adequate preload that is accompanied by systemic hypoperfusion. Specific clinical and hemodynamic criteria for cardiogenic shock caused by AMI are listed in **Box 1**.[2] Progressive end-organ dysfunction is a hallmark of persistent cardiogenic shock and necessitates intervention to overcome the altered hemodynamics and to restore end-organ perfusion. Vasopressors and positive inotropic agents act as the first lines of therapy, but often offer insufficient support. MCS devices such as durable left ventricular assist devices (LVADs) require surgical placement for which many patients are deemed too ill. Moreover, unstable patients with critical cardiogenic shock who receive a durable LVAD carry the highest postoperative mortality risk.[3]

Clinical studies that have examined cardiogenic shock have predominately focused on the high-risk PCI or AMI conditions (**Table 1**). However, shock can complicate many other conditions (**Box 2**), including chronic progressive heart failure.[12] The International Society of Heart and

Disclosures: The authors have nothing to disclose.
[a] Houston Methodist Hospital, 6550 Fannin Street, Suite 1901, Houston, TX 77030, USA; [b] Heart Transplant & LVAD Program, Division of Heart Failure, Houston Methodist Institute of Academic Medicine, Methodist DeBakey Heart & Vascular Center, Houston Methodist Hospital, 6550 Fannin Street, Suite 1901, Houston, TX 77030, USA
* Corresponding author.
E-mail address: jestep@houstonmethodist.org

Heart Failure Clin 12 (2016) 385–398
http://dx.doi.org/10.1016/j.hfc.2016.03.003
1551-7136/16/$ – see front matter © 2016 Elsevier Inc. All rights reserved.

Box 1
Cardiogenic shock[a] definition used in the SHOCK trial

Clinical criteria

- Hypotension:
  - Systolic blood pressure (SBP) less than 90 mm Hg for at least 30 minutes or
  - Need for supportive measures to maintain an SBP greater than or equal to 90 mm Hg
- End-organ hypoperfusion:
  - Cool extremities or
  - Urine output less than 30 mL/h and
  - Heart rate greater than 60 beats/min

Hemodynamic criteria

- Cardiac index less than or equal to 2.2 L/min/m² and
- Pulmonary capillary wedge pressure greater than or equal to 15 mm Hg

[a] Early revascularization in AMI complicated by cardiogenic shock.
Adapted from Hochman JS, Sleeper LA, Webb JG, et al. Early revascularization in acute myocardial infarction complicated by cardiogenic shock. SHOCK Investigators. Should We Emergently Revascularize Occluded Coronaries for Cardiogenic Shock. N Engl J Med 1999;341:626.

Lung Transplantation (ISHLT) 2013 guidelines recommend nondurable (temporary) MCS for acute decompensated heart failure failing maximal medical therapy, multiorgan failure, sepsis, or ventilator-dependent patients to optimize hemodynamics and evaluate neurologic status (class 1 recommendation).[13] More recently, a consensus summary statement including endorsement by the American Heart Association suggested several indications for percutaneous MCS (**Table 2**).[14] Percutaneous MCS devices can be placed emergently to unload the left ventricle, decrease intracardiac filling pressures and left ventricle volume, and provide increased cardiac output to restore vital organ perfusion. Given the dire consequences of systemic hypoperfusion in the setting of progressive cardiac dysfunction, the use of percutaneous MCS in severe, refractory cardiogenic shock should be considered early in a patient's clinical course. The use of temporary MCS devices has increased dramatically over the last few years. As noted by Stretch and colleagues,[15] their use in the United States alone has increased by more than 1000%, with percutaneous devices showing the fastest rate of growth among all forms of

MCS. These percutaneous MCS devices act as a bridge for critically ill patients, whether it is to recovery, durable mechanical support, or cardiac transplantation. **Fig. 1** shows the strategic role of temporary MCS, including patient and programmatic considerations.

The choice of which MCS device to use is based on many factors, including patient characteristics, the degree of desired hemodynamic support, operator abilities, and institutional resources. **Table 3** outlines the different characteristics of the available percutaneous devices. Although it offers the least amount of hemodynamic support, the intra-aortic balloon counterpulsation (intra-aortic balloon pump [IABP]) is widely available and most easily inserted during emergent bedside situations. However, several studies have shown that percutaneous MCS, including the Impella devices, TandemHeart, and veno-arterial extracorporeal membrane oxygenation (ECMO), provides greater hemodynamic support compared with IABP. This article provides an update on the types of percutaneous devices, hemodynamic effects, indications and contraindications for use, and management considerations for use in patients with cardiogenic shock.

TEMPORARY PERCUTANEOUS DEVICE TYPES AND HEMODYNAMIC EFFECTS

The device types described here are illustrated in **Fig. 2**. These devices can improve cardiac index, systemic blood pressure, and tissue perfusion to different degrees. In general, there is a continuum of increasing hemodynamic support from the IABP to the Impella 2.5 and CP devices to the TandemHeart and veno-arterial (VA) ECMO. This increased hemodynamic support is, in general terms, at the expense of more invasive vascular access and greater complication rates (bleeding and leg ischemia). The hemodynamic effects of percutaneous MCS in patients with cardiogenic shock are best understood through the effects of device support on the position and shape of the ventricular pressure-volume loop (PVL). As recently reviewed in the clinical consensus expert statement on percutaneous MCS[14] and by Burkhoff and colleagues,[16] many factors affect these PVLs. The anticipated patient response to percutaneous MCS also depends on the presenting clinical syndrome (ie, acute insult like myocardial infarction [MI] or acute on chronic left ventricular [LV] remodeling and/or right ventricular [RV] involvement). The response to percutaneous MCS must take into account underlying preload, afterload, LV contractility, and

Table 1
Selected clinical studies examining cardiogenic shock and percutaneous MCS

Selected Device Trials	Trial Type	Indication	Sample Size	Primary End Point	Result
IABP					
BCIS-1[4]	Randomized Elective IABP vs medical	High-risk PCI	N = 301	MACCE[a]	No difference (15.2% IABP vs 16% medical; P = .85)
Shock II trial[5]	Randomized IABP vs medical	AMI with cardiogenic shock	N = 600	30-d all-cause mortality	No difference (39.7% IABP vs 41.3% medical; P = .69)
Impella					
ISAR shock[6]	Randomized Impella 2.5 vs IABP	Cardiogenic shock	N = 25	Change of CI from baseline to 30 min	Difference seen (Impella CI change = 0.49 ± 0.46 L/min/m²; IABP change CI = 0.11 ± 0.31 L/min/m²; P = .02)
Protect II trial[7]	Randomized Impella 2.5 vs IABP	High-risk PCI[b]	N = 452	30-d incidence of major adverse events	No difference (35.1% for Impella vs 40.1% for IABP; P = .22)
RECOVER-I[8]	Nonrandomized prospective single arm (Impella 5.0)	Postcardiotomy shock	N = 16	30-d death or stroke survival to implantation of next therapy	13% stroke or death, 7% bridge to other therapy, and survival to 30 d was 94%
Recover Right trial[9]	Nonrandomized prospective single arm (Impella RP)	RV failure within 48 h post-LVAD, postcardiotomy, or MI shock	N = 30	30-d survival, hospital discharge, or bridge to next therapy	Difference seen 73% for Impella RP vs 58.3% benchmark reference[c]
Tandem Heart					
TandemHeart Trial[10]	Randomized TandemHeart vs IABP	AMI with cardiogenic shock	N = 41	Cardiac power index within 2 h after device placement	Difference seen (Tandem Heart CPI change from 0.22 to 0.37 W/m² compared with IABP from 0.22 to 28 W/m²; P = .004 intergroup comparison)
TandemHeart vs IABP[11]	Randomized TandemHeart vs IABP	Cardiogenic Shock	N = 42	Superior hemodynamic benefit	Difference seen greater decrease in PCWP and increase in CI and mean BP (TandemHeart vs IABP)

Abbreviations: BP, blood pressure; CI, cardiac index; CPI, Cardiac Power Index, calculated as product of cardiac index (CI) multiplied by mean arterial pressure (MAP) multiplied by 0.0022; MACCE, major adverse cardiovascular and cerebrovascular events; MI, myocardial infarction; PCWP, pulmonary capillary wedge pressure; RV, right ventricular; SHOCK trial, Should We Emergently Revascularize Occluded Coronaries for Cardiogenic Shock trial.
[a] MACCE defined as death, AMI, cerebrovascular event, or further revascularization at hospital discharge (capped at 28 days).
[b] Nonemergent symptomatic patients with complex 3-vessel disease or unprotected left main coronary artery disease and severely depressed LV function.
[c] Surgical HDE (Humanitarian Device Exception)-approved right ventricular assist device.
Adapted from Werdan K, Gielen S, Ebelt H, et al. Mechanical circulatory support in cardiogenic shock. Eur Heart J 2014;35:156-67.

Box 2
Causes of cardiogenic shock

- AMI and mechanical complications:
  - Left ventricular (LV) dysfunction
  - Right ventricular infarction
  - Acute mitral regurgitation
  - Ventricular septal defect
  - Pericardial tamponade
  - LV free wall rupture
- Acute ventricular failure:
  - Myocarditis
  - Transplant allograft rejection
  - Rapidly progressive dilated cardiomyopathy
  - Stress cardiomyopathy (Takotsubo)
  - Ventricular assist device dysfunction
- Acute on chronic progressive heart failure
- Valvular disorders:
  - Acute mitral regurgitation
  - Acute aortic regurgitation
  - Critical aortic stenosis
- Others:
  - After cardiac surgery
  - Septic shock with LV dysfunction
  - Pulmonary embolism
  - Myocardial contusion

Adapted from Doll JA, Ohman EM, Patel MR, et al. A team-based approach to patients in cardiogenic shock. Catheter Cardiovasc Interv 2015. [Epub ahead of print].

the pump speed (this influences flow) of the temporary device.

Intra-aortic Balloon Pump

The IABP comprises a 7.0-Fr to 8.0 Fr double-lumen catheter with a cylindrical polyethylene balloon that is advanced through an introducer sheath into the aorta. The device is synced with either the electrocardiogram or a pressure trigger for proper timing. The IABP rapidly shuttles helium gas in and out of the balloon located in the descending aorta. The balloon is inflated at the onset of cardiac diastole and augments pulsatile blood flow, which displaces blood volume in the descending aorta, resulting in increased mean aortic pressure and coronary perfusion pressure. The balloon deflates at the onset of systole, producing a vacuum effect that

decreases afterload and augments cardiac output. Optimal IABP function increases diastolic aortic pressure and reduces peak LV systolic and diastolic pressure and volume. LV stroke volume is mildly increased with IABP support. The net hemodynamic effect is reduced effective arterial elastance, a component of LV afterload defined as the ratio of end-systolic pressure (decreased with IABP) and stoke volume (increased with IABP) (**Fig. 3**).

The IABP controller console displays a pressure waveform that is used to assess the degree of hemodynamic support, or blood pressure augmentation, as well as the timing of the device. The choice of frequency of IABP inflation for each cardiac cycle depends on the degree of augmentation desired, with the most frequent setting being 1:1. Larger capacity IABPs (eg, 50 cc) potentially offer greater hemodynamic support (greater diastolic augmentation and systolic unloading) than the standard 40 cc IABP.[17,18] However, there remains a paucity of data limited to acute MI-related cardiogenic shock that defines the degree of hemodynamic benefit provided by the IABP (see **Table 1**). To our knowledge there are no clinical studies that have examined the clinical benefits (including hemodynamics) and risks of IABP therapy in patients with advanced heart failure and cardiogenic shock not related to AMI or high-risk PCI.

All percutaneous MCS devices require full anticoagulation. Specifically, for patients with IABP support anticoagulation is recommended to prevent thrombus formation on the balloon; however, in patients with a high risk of bleeding or active bleeding, the IABP can be used for a short time at a 1:1 setting without anticoagulation. The IABP can be removed at the bedside and hemostasis achieved with manual pressure. Because the IABP sits in the proximal aorta and provides counterpulsation during ventricular diastole, the device is contraindicated in patients with greater than mild aortic regurgitation (see **Table 3**). Severe peripheral arterial disease also precludes the use of this device because of the risk of vascular complications and limb ischemia. Of note, the IABP is traditionally placed via femoral arterial access, but it can also be placed in the left axillary artery to allow the patient to sit up and ambulate. This location offers the patient greater mobility and has been shown to be effective in patients requiring mechanical support while awaiting cardiac transplant.[19] A limitation of the IABP is its dependence on native LV contractility and modest effect on cardiac output, points that are paramount when deciding which MCS device to use in a given clinical situation.

Table 2
Suggested indications for percutaneous MCS

Indication	Comments
Complications of AMI	Ischemic mitral regurgitation is particularly well suited to these devices because the hemodynamic disturbance is usually acute and substantial. Acutely depressed LV function from large AMIs during and after primary PCI is an increasing indication for temporary MCS use. Cardiogenic shock from RV infarction can be treated with percutaneous RV support
Severe heart failure in the setting of nonischemic cardiomyopathy	Examples include severe exacerbations of chronic systolic heart failure as well as acutely reversible cardiomyopathies such as fulminant myocarditis, stress cardiomyopathy, or peripartum cardiomyopathy. In patients presenting in INTERMACS profiles 1 or 2, MCS can be used as a bridge to destination VAD placement or as a bridge to recovery if the ejection fraction rapidly improves
Acute cardiac allograft failure	Primary allograft failure (adult or pediatric) may be caused by acute cellular or antibody-mediated rejection, prolonged ischemic time, or inadequate organ preservation
Posttransplant RV failure	Acute RV failure has several potential causes, including recipient pulmonary hypertension, intraoperative injury/ischemia, and excess volume/blood product resuscitation. MCS support provides time for the donor right ventricle to recover function, often with the assistance of inotropic and pulmonary vasodilator therapy
Patients slow to wean from cardiopulmonary bypass following heart surgery	Although selected patients may be transitioned to a percutaneous system for additional weaning, this is rarely done
Refractory arrhythmias	Patients can be treated with a percutaneous system that is somewhat independent of the cardiac rhythm. For recurrent, refractory ventricular arrhythmias, ECMO may be required for biventricular failure
Prophylactic use for high-risk PCI	Particularly in patients with severe LV dysfunction (EF <20%–30%) and complex coronary artery disease involving a large territory (sole remaining vessel, left main or 3-vessel disease)
High-risk or complex ablation of VT	Similar to high-risk PCI, complex VT ablation can be made feasible with percutaneous support. MCS use allows the patient to remain in VT longer during arrhythmia mapping without as much concern about systemic hypoperfusion
High-risk percutaneous valve interventions	These evolving procedures may be aided with the use of MCSs

Abbreviations: EF, ejection fraction; INTERMACS, interagency registry for mechanically assisted circulatory support; LV, left ventricular; VAD, ventricular assist device; VT, ventricular tachycardia.

Adapted from Rihal CS, Naidu SS, Givertz MM, et al. 2015 SCAI/ACC/HFSA/STS Clinical expert consensus statement on the use of percutaneous mechanical circulatory support devices in cardiovascular care. J Am Coll Cardiol 2015;65:e18; with permission.

Impella Circulatory Support System

The Impella (Abiomed; Danvers, MA) is an axial flow pump containing an Archimedes screw impeller attached to a catheter with a pigtail tip designed to sit in the LV. When inserted into the femoral artery via the appropriate-sized introducer sheath and advanced retrograde across the aortic valve, the device draws blood from the LV via an inlet area through the impeller and into the ascending aorta via an outlet area proximal to the pigtail (**Fig. 4**). There are currently 3 left-sided

Impella support devices available that offer differing degrees of hemodynamic support based on size: the Impella 2.5, which has a 9-Fr catheter attached to a 12-Fr motor that can provide up to 2.5 L/min flow; the Impella CP with a 9-Fr catheter attached to a 14-Fr motor that can provide up to 4 L/min flow, and the Impella 5.0 with a 9-Fr catheter attached to a 21-Fr motor that can provide up to 5 L/min flow. The 2.5 and CP devices are generally placed via femoral arterial access, as described earlier, and come with an introducer sheath that corresponds to the motor size.

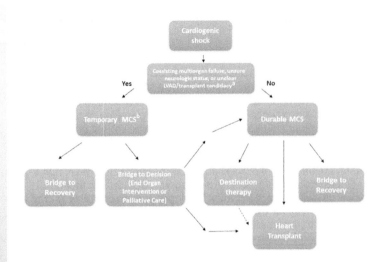

Fig. 1. Role of temporary MCS and patient and programmatic considerations. [a] Based on institution's programmatic inclusion and exclusion criteria. [b] Includes percutaneous device options.

However, given its size, the Impella 5.0 requires a surgical cutdown and is frequently placed in the axillary artery via a vascular graft through a 23-Fr introducer sheath.

As shown by the PVLs, continuous augmented flow of blood independent of the cardiac cycle directly from the left ventricle results in loss of the normal isovolumic periods, which transforms the shape of the PVL from the normal trapezoidal to a triangular shape and therefore, as the pump speed is increased (eg, P2 to P8 to augment flow from 1.5 to 4.5 L/min), the PVL shifts leftward and the net hemodynamic effect is a decrease in peak LV pressure generation and volume, along with marked decreases in the pressure-volume area and myocardial oxygen consumption (MVO2) (see **Fig. 3**). The main hemodynamic effect is a reduction in LV end-diastolic pressure (LVEDP) as arterial pressure increases, and as the LV stroke volume decreases the peak LV pressure and arterial pressure become increasingly dissociated.[16]

The pump improves the hemodynamics associated with cardiogenic shock by unloading the left ventricle, resulting in an increased mean arterial pressure (MAP) and reduced myocardial oxygen demand and pulmonary capillary wedge pressure (PCWP). Based on ISAR-Shock (A Randomized Clinical Trial to Evaluate the Safety and Efficacy of a Percutaneous Left Ventricular Assist Device Versus Intra-Aortic Balloon Pumping for Treatment of Cardiogenic Shock Caused by Myocardial Infarction), the Impella 2.5 LP device increased cardiac index greater than the IABP (0.49 ± 0.46 L/min/m^2 compared with a change of 0.11 ± 0.31 L/min/m^2; $P<.01$).[6] To our knowledge there are no human studies that define the hemodynamic effects of the Impella CP device. Two preclinical studies have shown that, with the

larger Impella device platforms (eg, Impella CP), 3.1 to 3.8 L/min of flow can be generated and LV stroke work reduced by ~32% to 50%. There is only 1 prospective study that examined the hemodynamic effects of the Impella 5.0 device. In the RECOVER-I (multicenter prospective study of Impella 5.0/LD for postcardiotomy circulatory support) trial,[8] the Impella 5.0 significantly increased cardiac index from 1.65 to 2.7 L/min/m^2, MAP increased from 71 to 83 mm Hg, and pulmonary diastolic pressure decreased from 29 to 20 mm Hg (see **Table 1**).

Proper positioning of the Impella within the left ventricle is key to optimizing support. Although it is initially positioned using fluoroscopy, most commonly in the catheterization laboratory, echocardiography is the imaging modality of choice to identify proper positioning at the patient's bedside (**Fig. 5**). If the device sits too high in the LV outflow tract there is a risk of the distal pigtail catheter prolapsing back across the aortic valve into the ascending aorta and thus resulting in no LV support. In contrast, if the catheter is advanced too far into the LV apex there is a risk of ventricular arrhythmias and perforation. An Impella device that sits too deep in the LV cavity can also result in an outlet area positioned below the aortic valve, which provides no LV support or augmentation of cardiac output. There is also a significant increase in hemolysis when the device is malpositioned. Note that because the Impella device sits within the LV, there can be instances of LV suction in which the left ventricle size is reduced sufficiently for the ventricular wall to contact the catheter. This phenomenon occurs in the setting of LV underfilling, and is caused by a significant reduction in LV preload, such as in instances of RV failure or hypovolemia.[20]

However, cardiogenic shock does not always occur in the context of LV failure alone, but can come in the form of severe RV dysfunction or biventricular failure. Furthermore, initiating LV support (with a temporary percutaneous device or durable LVAD) in the setting of a tenuous right ventricle can induce fulminant RV failure necessitating RV MCS. The newest device in the Impella family, the Impella RP, provides RV support in patients who develop RV failure after myocardial infarction or after cardiotomy following LVAD implantation or cardiac transplant.[9] The pump is composed of an 11-Fr catheter attached to a 22-Fr motor that can provide up to 4 L/min flow. The inlet area sits in the inferior vena cava, with the outlet at the tip of the catheter, which is positioned in the pulmonary artery (**Fig. 6**A). This device can be used alone in the case of isolated RV failure, or in conjunction with left-sided MCS support devices for biventricular support (**Fig. 6**B).

Tandem Heart Percutaneous Ventricular Assist Device System

The TandemHeart percutaneous ventricular assist device (Cardiac Assist, Inc; Pittsburgh, PA) is an extracorporeal left atrium to femoral artery bypass continuous flow centrifugal pump that can provide support of up to 4 L/min. A 21-Fr inflow cannula whose distal portion contains 14 side holes and a large end hole is placed in the femoral artery and advanced via transseptal puncture into the left atrium, where oxygenated blood is then removed and pumped into the abdominal aorta via a 15-Fr to 17-Fr outflow cannula inserted into the contralateral femoral artery (see **Fig. 2**; **Fig. 7**). There is a paucity of studies examining the hemodynamic effects of the TandemHeart, but the device has been shown to increase cardiac output and provide volume unloading of the left ventricle, overall resulting in a decrease in PCWP, central venous pressure, and pulmonary artery pressure; and reduced biventricular filling pressures, cardiac workload, and oxygen demand.[11,21] The net flow-dependent effect of the TandemHeart is reduction in end-diastolic pressures and native LV stroke volume and an increase in end-systolic volume (see **Fig. 3**).

Given the large cannula size, limb ischemia distal to the insertion site is a significant concern, and an antegrade sheath can be placed in the superficial femoral artery (SFA) and connected to the outflow cannula to provide improved limb perfusion. Full anticoagulation is recommended to prevent thrombotic complications. The TandemHeart requires some degree of RV function to maintain necessary left atrial volume, although, in the setting of progressive RV failure, the device can be converted to an ECMO circuit by repositioning the inflow cannula back across the interatrial septum into the right atrium and a membrane oxygenator added to the circuit to provide biventricular support. Kapur and colleagues[22] also described the successful use of the TandemHeart as a centrifugal flow–RV support device in instances of RV failure. This percutaneous MCS device has been shown to significantly improve rates of survival to durable LVAD or transplantation,[21,23] and thus should be considered in patients with refractory cardiogenic shock.

Extracorporeal Membrane Oxygenation

There are 2 varieties of extracorporeal support, based on the degree of hemodynamic compromise. The venoveno system is used solely for oxygenation support, such as in adult respiratory distress syndrome. However, the veno-arterial system provides total cardiopulmonary and biventricular support, with augmentation of cardiac output and MAP. The components include a continuous flow pump for blood propulsion and a membrane oxygenator for gas exchange. In VA ECMO, a venous inflow cannula (sizes ranging from 15 to 29 Fr) is placed in the femoral vein and advanced into the right atrium, where deoxygenated blood is aspirated and circulated via a centrifugal pump through a membrane oxygenator. The oxygenated blood is then pumped into the abdominal aorta via an arterial outflow cannula (sizes ranging from 15 to 23 Fr) that is inserted into the femoral artery (see **Fig. 2**). VA ECMO can provide flows up to 6 L/min and the degree of support depends on the cannula sizes.

The primary hemodynamic effect of such right atrium to arterial circulatory support is increased LV afterload and effective arterial elastance. As shown in **Fig. 3**, as ECMO flow is increased, total peripheral resistance and LV contractility are not changed. The LV response to increased LV afterload is blood accumulation in the LV. The adverse consequence in patients with cardiogenic shock is a subsequent increase in LVEDP and PCWP and the native LV stroke volume becomes increasingly small.[14,16] These negative consequences may exacerbate the congestive state unless the left ventricle is unloaded or vented. LV decompression strategies with VA ECMO include percutaneous options (IABP, Impella, transseptal left atrial cannulation, atrial septostomy); surgery (direct LV apical or left atrial cannulation); or noninvasive optimization, including inotropic support. Eventually it may be necessary to reduce the VA ECMO.[14,20,24,25]

Table 3
Selected temporary MCS device types and characteristics

Device	Type of Pump	Indication	Vascular Access	Contraindications	Complications/Challenges
IABP	Pulsatile, pneumatic	Cardiogenic shock AMI mechanical complication Weaning from cardiopulmonary bypass High-risk PCI Complications of HF, ischemic and nonischemic	Arterial; femoral or left axillary/subclavian	Severe peripheral vascular disease Moderate or worse aortic insufficiency Aortic dissection Abdominal aortic aneurysm Contraindication to anticoagulation	Aortic dissection or rupture Renal or bowel ischemia if incorrect positioning Unstable arrhythmias if axillary IABP repositions into left ventricle Bleeding Limb ischemia
Impella 2.5	Continuous axial flow, Archimedes screw impeller	High-risk intervention	Arterial; femoral	Aortic valve stenosis (AVA $\leq$0.6 cm^2) Mechanical aortic valve Severe peripheral vascular disease Moderate or worse aortic insufficiency Mural LV thrombus Contraindication to anticoagulation	Aortic valve injury Migration of the pigtail back across the aortic valve Ventricular arrhythmias caused by malposition Hemolysis Pump thrombosis Tamponade caused by LV perforation Bleeding Limb ischemia Stroke
Impella CP	Continuous axial flow, Archimedes screw impeller	Partial circulatory support	Arterial; femoral	As above	As above
Impella 5.0[a,b]	Continuous axial flow, Archimedes screw impeller	Circulatory support	Arterial; femoral or axillary[a]	As above, with the exception of peripheral vascular disease for axillary access	As above, with the exception of limb ischemia for axillary access

Impella RP	Continuous axial flow, Archimedes screw impeller	Right ventricular failure (MI, post-LVAD, heart transplant or postcardiotomy)	Venous; internal jugular	Mechanical tricuspid or pulmonic valves Right atrial or IVC thrombus Severe tricuspid or pulmonic stenosis Presence of IVC filter that cannot accommodate 22-F sheath Contraindication to anticoagulation	Small ventricular cavity
TandemHeart	Continuous flow, centrifugal	Cardiogenic shock, cleared for use with an oxygenator	Arterial and venous; femoral	Severe peripheral vascular disease Right or left atrial thrombus Ventricular septal defect Contraindication to anticoagulation	Migration of the inflow cannula into the right atrium causing massive shunt Migration of the inflow cannula into the pulmonary vein causing pump malfunction Tamponade caused by atrial perforation Creation of atrial septal defect Pump thrombosis Bleeding Limb ischemia Stroke
VA ECMO	Continuous flow, centrifugal	Cardiogenic shock with impaired oxygenation	Arterial and venous; femoral	Severe peripheral vascular disease Right atrial thrombus Contraindication to anticoagulation	Differential oxygenation (*harlequin syndrome*) Pump thrombosis Bleeding Limb ischemia

Abbreviations: AVA, aortic valve area; HF, heart failure; IABP, intra-aortic balloon pump; IVC, inferior vena cava; VA, veno-arterial.

a Requires a surgical cutdown.

b Requires a Dacron vascular graft, 10 mm recommended size.

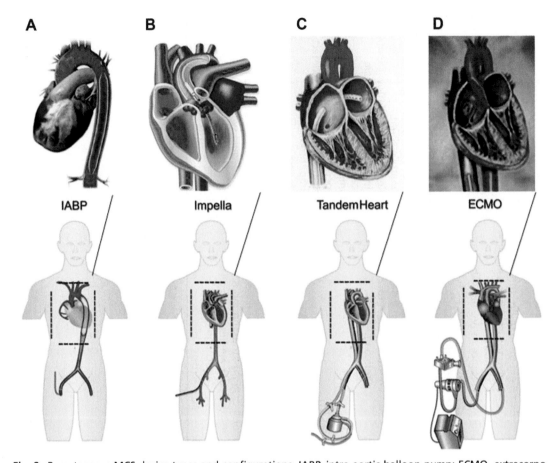

Fig. 2. Percutaneous MCS device types and configurations. IABP, intra aortic balloon pump; ECMO, extracorporeal membrane oxygenation. (*Adapted from* Werdan K, Gielen S, Ebelt H, et al. Mechanical circulatory support in cardiogenic shock. Eur Heart J 2014;35:156–67; and Thiele H, Zeymer U, Neumann FJ, et al. Intra-aortic balloon counterpulsation in acute myocardial infarction complicated by cardiogenic shock (IABP-SHOCK II): final 12 month results of a randomised, open-label trial. Lancet 2013;382:160; with permission.)

Of note, there is a distinct clinical scenario that sometimes complicates ECMO support. LV recovery during VA ECMO support can produce competitive flow in the aorta, resulting in desaturated blood perfusing the head and upper extremities (blue head) while oxygenated blood is directed to the lower extremities (red legs). A femoral IABP proximal to the ECMO outflow cannula can also result in this phenomenon, occasionally referred to as the harlequin syndrome.[20,26] Clinicians can monitor for this syndrome and detect it in the early stages by measuring pulse oximetry and occasional arterial blood gas measurements in the right arm, while monitoring for LV recovery with surveillance echocardiography.

There are no randomized studies comparing VA ECMO with other percutaneous MCS therapies. Cheng and colleagues[27] recently performed a meta-analysis of 20 studies including 1866 patients with cardiac arrest or cardiogenic shock.

Based on their analysis, complications were common, including major or significant bleeding (41.9%), lower extremity ischemia (16.9%), fasciotomy or compartment syndrome (10.3%), and stroke (5.9%). In an effort to minimize distal limb ischemia in the setting of such large cannulas, an antegrade sheath can be placed in the SFA and connected to the arterial cannula to provide improved distal limb perfusion.[28]

THE CARDIOGENIC SHOCK TEAM

Several centers, in addition to the recent expert consensus on the use of percutaneous MCS, endorse a team approach with input from an advanced heart failure cardiologist, interventional cardiologist, cardiac intensivist, and cardiothoracic surgeon.[12,14,29,30] The organization and primary function of the cardiogenic shock team is to coordinate physician activation, discuss and

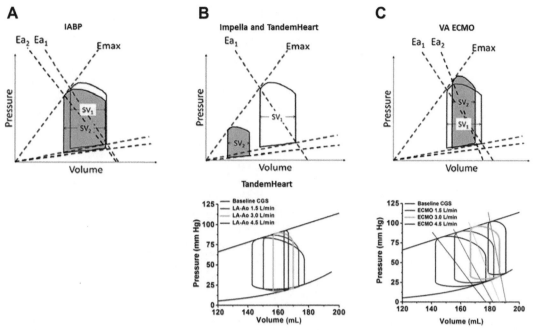

Fig. 3. Hemodynamic effects of the different percutaneous MCS device types. (*A*) IABP counterpulsation reduces peak LV systolic and diastolic pressures and increases LV stroke volume. The net effect is a reduced slope of arterial elastance (Ea$_2$). (*B*) Upper panel shows Impella and TandemHeart with significantly reduced LV pressures, LV volumes, and LV stroke volume. The net effect is significant reduction in cardiac workload. Lower panel shows flow-dependent changes in the PVL with TandemHeart left atrium–aorta (LA–Ao) support showing reduced end-diastolic pressures, increased end-systolic volume, and decreased LV stroke volume with increased pump flow from 1.5 to 4.5 L/min. (*C*) Upper panel shows that VA ECMO without LV venting increases LV systolic and diastolic pressure and reduces LV stroke volume with a net effect of increased arterial Ea$_2$. Lower panel shows the impact of flow-dependent increases in VA ECMO support (1.5–4.5 L/min) with increasing end-diastolic pressures, increases of effective arterial elastance, and decreases in LV stroke volume. CGS, cardiogenic shock; Ea1, effective arterial elastance; SV1, stroke volume in condition 1; SV2, stroke volume in condition 2. (*Adapted from* Rihal CS, Naidu SS, Givertz MM, et al. 2015 SCAI/ACC/HFSA/STS Clinical expert consensus statement on the use of percutaneous mechanical circulatory support devices in cardiovascular care. J Am Coll Cardiol 2015;65:e10; and Burkhoff D, Sayer G, Doshi D, et al. Hemodynamics of Mechanical Circulatory Support. J Am Coll Cardiol 2015;66:2669; with permission.)

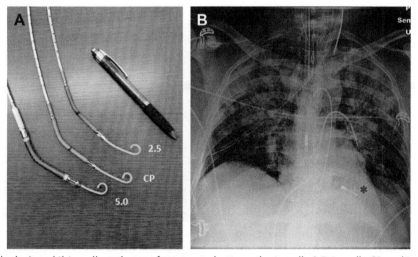

Fig. 4. Impella devices. (*A*) Impella catheters; from top to bottom, the Impella 2.5, Impella CP, and Impella 5.0. (*B*) Proper Impella position (*red asterisk*) seen on chest radiograph.

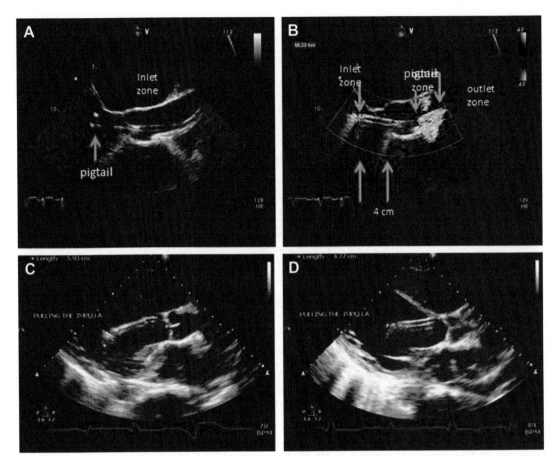

Fig. 5. Impella positioning using echocardiography. (*A*) Transesophageal echocardiography (TEE) image showing Impella sitting too high in the LV outflow tract, with the device inlet zone above the aortic valve. (*B*) TEE image following Impella repositioning (advanced further into the LV), with the inlet zone 4 cm below the aortic valve (goal ∼3–4 cm). (*C*) TTE image showing the Impella device sitting too deep in the LV. In this instance, the device can be withdrawn a few centimeters and position reassessed (*D*).

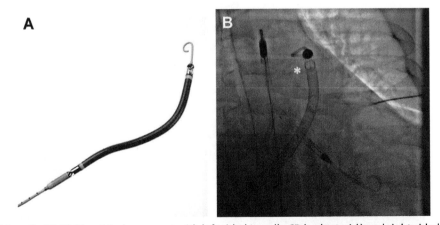

Fig. 6. (*A*) Impella RP. (*B*) Biventricular support with left-sided Impella CP (*red asterisk*) and right-sided Impella RP (*yellow asterisk*). ([A] *From* Cheung AW, White CW, Davis MK, et al. Short-term mechanical circulatory support for recovery from acute right ventricular failure: clinical outcomes. J Heart Lung Transplant 2014;33:795; with permission; and [B] *Courtesy of* B. Aertker, MD, Houston, TX.)

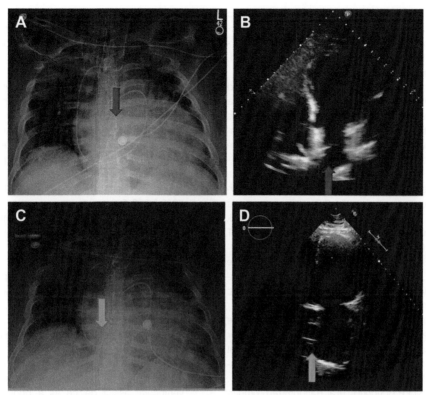

Fig. 7. TandemHeart positioning. Chest radiograph (*A*) and transthoracic echocardiogram (*B*) showing proper TandemHeart inflow cannula position across the interatrial septum with the distal tip in the left atrium (*red arrows*), compared with a chest radiograph (*C*) and transthoracic echocardiogram (*D*) showing inflow cannula malposition with the distal tip in the right atrium (*blue arrows*). Of note, at the time of malposition, there is only venous blood visualized in the TandemHeart system.

organize escalation of necessary services (eg, emergent revascularization), promote early transfer to an LVAD/transplant center, and address deactivation of therapies when cardiogenic shock resolves, durable LVAD or heart transplantation takes place, or if there is a transition to comfort care.[12] The observations made based on a team approach show proof of concept and feasibility. However, the effectiveness and benefits of this multidisciplinary team approach remain to be determined.

SUMMARY

Cardiogenic shock, as a result of acute insult or severe decompensation of chronic heart failure, is often associated with rapidly progressive multiorgan dysfunction caused by systemic hypoperfusion. Temporary mechanical circulatory support devices, specifically those placed percutaneously, provide a means of restoring perfusion to allow for recovery or eventual long-term MCS or transplant. As described earlier, there are several options for temporary percutaneous MCS, each offering

variable degrees of hemodynamic support. The choice of which device to use is multifactorial, and these devices are best managed with a team approach.

REFERENCES

1. Levine GN, Bates ER, Blankenship JC, et al. 2011 ACCF/AHA/SCAI guideline for percutaneous coronary intervention. J Am Coll Cardiol 2011;58:e44–122.
2. Hochman JS, Sleeper LA, Webb JG, et al. Early revascularization in acute myocardial infarction complicated by cardiogenic shock. SHOCK investigators. Should we emergently revascularize occluded coronaries for cardiogenic shock. N Engl J Med 1999;341:625–34.
3. Kirklin JK, Naftel DC, Pagani FD, et al. Sixth INTERMACS annual report: a 10,000-patient database. J Heart Lung Transplant 2014;33:555–64.
4. Perera D, Stables R, Thomas M, et al, BCIS-1 Investigators. Elective intra-aortic balloon counterpulsation during high-risk percutaneous coronary intervention: a randomized controlled trial. JAMA 2010;304:867–74.

5. Thiele H, Zeymer U, Neumann FJ, et al. Intra-aortic balloon counterpulsation in acute myocardial infarction complicated by cardiogenic shock (IABP-SHOCK II): final 12 month results of a randomised, open-label trial. Lancet 2013;382:1638–45.

6. Seyfarth M, Sibbing D, Bauer I, et al. A randomized clinical trial to evaluate the safety and efficacy of a percutaneous left ventricular assist device versus intra-aortic balloon pumping for treatment of cardiogenic shock caused by myocardial infarction. J Am Coll Cardiol 2008;52:1584–8.

7. O'Neill WW, Kleiman NS, Moses J, et al. A prospective, randomized clinical trial of hemodynamic support with Impella 2.5 versus intra-aortic balloon pump in patients undergoing high-risk percutaneous coronary intervention: the PROTECT II study. Circulation 2012;126:1717–27.

8. Griffith BP, Anderson MB, Samuels LE, et al. The RECOVER I: a multicenter prospective study of Impella 5.0/LD for postcardiotomy circulatory support. J Thorac Cardiovasc Surg 2013;145:548–54.

9. Anderson MB, Goldstein J, Milano C, et al. Benefits of a novel percutaneous ventricular assist device for right heart failure: the prospective recover right study of the Impella RP device. J Heart Lung Transplant 2015;34:1549–60.

10. Thiele H, Sick P, Boudriot E, et al. Randomized comparison of intra-aortic balloon support with a percutaneous left ventricular assist device in patients with revascularized acute myocardial infarction complicated by cardiogenic shock. Eur Heart J 2005;26:1276–83.

11. Burkhoff D, Cohen H, Brunckhorst C, et al, TandemHeart Investigators Group, TandemHeart Investigators Group. A randomized multicenter clinical study to evaluate the safety and efficacy of the TandemHeart percutaneous ventricular assist device vs conventional therapy with intraaortic balloon pumping for treatment of cardiogenic shock. Am Heart J 2006;152:469.e1–8.

12. Doll JA, Ohman EM, Patel MR, et al. A team-based approach to patients in cardiogenic shock. Catheter Cardiovasc Interv 2015. [Epub ahead of print].

13. Feldman D, Pamboukian SV, Teuteberg JJ, et al. The 2013 International Society for Heart and Lung Transplantation guidelines for mechanical circulatory support: executive summary. J Heart Lung Transplant 2013;32:157–87.

14. Rihal CS, Naidu SS, Givertz MM, et al. 2015 SCAI/ACC/HFSA/STS clinical expert consensus statement on the use of percutaneous mechanical circulatory support devices in cardiovascular care. J Am Coll Cardiol 2015;65:e7–26.

15. Stretch R, Sauer CM, Yuh DD, et al. National trends in the utilization of short-term mechanical circulatory support. J Am Coll Cardiol 2014;64:1407–15.

16. Burkhoff D, Sayer G, Doshi D, et al. Hemodynamics of mechanical circulatory support. J Am Coll Cardiol 2015;66:2663–74.

17. Majithia A, Jumean M, Shih H, et al. The hemodynamic effects of the MEGA intra-aortic balloon counterpulsation pump. J Heart Lung Transplant 2013; 32:S226.

18. Kapur NK, Paruchuri V, Majithia A, et al. Hemodynamic effects of standard versus larger-capacity intraaortic balloon counterpulsation pumps. J Invasive Cardiol 2015;27:182–8.

19. Estep J, Cordero-Reyes AM, Bhimaraj A, et al. Percutaneous placement of an intra-aortic balloon pump in the left axillary/subclavian position provides safe, ambulatory long-term support as bridge to heart transplantation. JACC Heart Fail 2013;5:382–8.

20. Lawson WE, Koo M. Percutaneous ventricular assist devices and ECMO in the management of acute decompensated heart failure. Clin Med Insights Cardiol 2015;9(Suppl 1):41–8.

21. Kar B, Gregoric ID, Basra SS, et al. The percutaneous ventricular assist device in severe refractory cardiogenic shock. J Am Coll Cardiol 2011;57:688–96.

22. Kapur NK, Paruchuri V, Jagannathan A, et al. Mechanical circulatory support for right ventricular failure. JACC Heart Fail 2013;1:127–34.

23. Bruckner BA, Jacob LP, Gregoric ID, et al. Clinical experience with the TandemHeart percutaneous ventricular assist device as a bridge to cardiac transplantation. Tex Heart Inst J 2008;35:447–50.

24. Kawashima D, Gojo S, Nishimura T, et al. Left ventricular mechanical support with Impella provides more ventricular unloading in heart failure than extracorporeal membrane oxygenation. ASAIO J 2011;57:169–76.

25. Koeckert MS, Jorde UP, Naka Y, et al. Impella LP 2.5 for left ventricular unloading during venoarterial extracorporeal membrane oxygenation support. J Card Surg 2011;26:666–8.

26. Rupprecht L, Lunz D, Philipp A, et al. Pitfalls in percutaneous ECMO cannulation. Heart Lung Vessel 2015;7(4):320–6.

27. Cheng R, Hachamovitch R, Kittleson M, et al. Complications of extracorporeal membrane oxygenation for treatment of cardiogenic shock and cardiac arrest: a meta-analysis of 1,866 adult patients. Ann Thorac Surg 2014;97(2):610–6.

28. Mohite PN, Fatullayev J, Maunz O, et al. Distal limb perfusion: Achilles' heel in peripheral venoarterial extracorporeal membrane oxygenation. Artif Organs 2014;38:940–4.

29. Burzotta F, Trani C, Doshi SN, et al. Impella ventricular support in clinical practice: collaborative viewpoint from a European expert user group. Int J Cardiol 2015;201:684–91.

30. Takayama H, Truby L, Koekort M, et al. Clinical outcome of mechanical circulatory support for refractory cardiogenic shock in the current era. J Heart Lung Transplant 2013;32:106–11.

Role of Durable Mechanical Circulatory Support for the Management of Advanced Heart Failure

Muhammed Waqas, MD, Jennifer A. Cowger, MD, MS*

KEYWORDS

- Mechanical circulatory support • Outcomes • Advanced heart failure management

KEY POINTS

- The number of patients with end-stage systolic heart failure (HF) managed with mechanical circulatory support (MCS) has increased more than 100% since 2009 but MCS remains an underused therapy.
- Current 1-year and 4-year average survival rates on MCS are 80% and approximately 50%, respectively, with higher survival in those supported for the bridge to transplant (BTT) indication.
- Early referral to an advanced HF specialist with MCS surgical capabilities is critical to ensure good outcomes for patients with recalcitrant HF (New York Heart Association [NYHA] classes III and IV).
- High-risk HF features include more than 1 admission in 6 months for HF, inability to tolerate guideline doses of HF medications due to hypotension, rising creatinine, escalating diuretic use and/or need for sequential nephron blockade, recurrent ventricular dysrhythmias, and signs of hepatic congestion (elevated international normalized ratio [INR] or bilirubin) and/or anorexia.

INTRODUCTION

HF is a major public health problem resulting in substantial morbidity, mortality, and health care expenditures. Currently there are an estimated 6 million Americans living with HF and this incidence is projected to rise substantially, with HF affecting an estimated 8 million individuals by 2030.[1] Of those with HF, an estimated 5% have end-stage (stage D) HF, recalcitrant to evidence-based medical therapy and/or biventricular pacing.[2]

Management options for advanced HF include MCS, cardiac transplant, inotrope support, and/or palliative care/hospice. Each management option carries its own associated survival expectancy (ranging from 25% to 90% at 1 year) and morbidity, and the care plan must be tailored to patients based on patient wishes and the ability to tolerate a major surgical procedure with acceptable morbidity and mortality. See Kittleson MM: Changing Role of Heart Transplantation; and Ginwalla M: Home Inotropes and Other Palliative Care, in this issue, other articles provide detailed reviews on the roles for cardiac transplant and palliative care/hospice for management of advanced HF. The focus in this article is on MCS.

ROLE OF MECHANICAL CIRCULATORY SUPPORT IN ADVANCE HEART FAILURE

Given strict cardiac transplant criteria and limited donor organ supply in the United States, the utilization of MCS for management of stage D HF has increased. More than 15,000 MCS implants

St. Vincent Heart Center of Indiana, Indianapolis, IN 46260, USA
* Corresponding author. Department of Advanced Heart Failure, 8333 Naab Road, Suite 400, Indianapolis, IN 46260.
E-mail address: jennifercowger@gmail.com

Heart Failure Clin 12 (2016) 399–409
http://dx.doi.org/10.1016/j.hfc.2016.03.012
1551-7136/16/$ – see front matter © 2016 Elsevier Inc. All rights reserved.

have been reported to the Interagency Registry for Mechanically Assisted Circulatory Support (INTERMACS), a database that collects outcomes on Food and Drug Administration (FDA)-approved durable MCS devices implanted within the United States.[3] Between 2009 and 2015, the number of MCS implants per year increased more than 100%, from 1000 to more than 2500 implants per year.[3] Although the number of patients supported with MCS is on the rise, MCS is still only applied to a minority of individuals with advanced HF. It is estimated that 150,000 individuals could benefit from MCS therapy in the United States.[4] The goal of this review is to educate practitioners on the types of MCS devices available for advanced HF, survival rates, complications associated with support, and the importance of timely referral for MCS evaluation.

CLASSIFYING MECHANICAL CIRCULATORY SUPPORT

There are a variety of FDA-approved and investigational circulatory pumps available in the United States. Most pumps are implanted with the aim of providing isolated left ventricle (LV) support as an LV assist device (LVAD). Patients with biventricular failure can be supported with biventricular mechanical support in form of a right ventricular assist device (RVAD) plus an LVAD, or via a total artificial heart. Durable RVAD support is not currently FDA approved. More than 612 durable and temporary RVADs (used in conjunction with LVAD support) have been reported to INTERMACS.[3] Total artificial heart support encompasses approximately 301 patients with stage D HF in INTERMACS and is currently approved for patients being supported with the goal for transplant.

MCS can also be classified based on duration of intended support (temporary vs durable), location of device implant (extracorporeal, intracorporeal, or paracorporeal), and device flow profile. Temporary devices are used for days to weeks and are used either as a bridge to myocardial recovery, cardiac transplant, or for eventual exchange to a permanent (also known as durable) MCS device. A detailed summary of temporary mechanical support and use of paracorporeal and extracorporeal devices is provided (see Brown JL, Estep, JD: Temporary Percutaneous Mechanical Circulatory Support in Advanced Heart Failure, in this issue).

Permanent/durable circulatory support devices are all intracorporeal in location. Devices vary on whether they provide continuous flow (CF) or pulsatile flow (**Table 1**). Currently in the United States, more than 90% of MCS patients are supported with a CF profile device. The remaining 10% of patients are largely supported with the pulsatile total artificial heart.[3] CF devices are further subcategorized as CF with axial-flow or CF with centrifugal-flow designs. In a typical CF device configuration, an inflow cannula delivers blood out the LV apex into a contained pump that then propels flood into the ascending aorta via a synthetic graft (**Fig. 1**). The current FDA-approved durable CF pumps are capable of providing up to 10 L of cardiac output.[5,6] Because flow is removed continuously from the LV during the cardiac cycle, intracavity LV pressures during isovolumic contraction often do not exceed aortic systolic pressure; hence, the aortic valve tends to remain closed during CF-LVAD support. As such, many patients on CF-LVAD support do not have a palpable peripheral pulse.

INDICATIONS FOR DEVICE SUPPORT IN THE UNITED STATES

In the United States, MCS devices are largely implanted for 1 of 2 payer-approved indications: as a bridge to cardiac transplant (BTT) or for permanent therapy (also known as destination therapy [DT]) without intent for future transplant. Predicting the postimplant trajectory of HF care prior to ventricular assist device [VAD] implantation is met with challenge, and the DT versus BTT designation for many individuals is payer-driven semantics. Patients who appear very ill pre-VAD can have dramatic functional and end-organ improvements after VAD and subsequently become fit for cardiac

Table 1 Clinically used left ventricular assist device types			
	First Generation	**Second Generation**	**Third Generation**
Pump design	Pulsatile flow	Continuous-flow (axial pump)	CF (centrifugal pump)
LVAD type	HeartMate IP1000, VE, XVE Novacor LVAD	HMII Incor Berlin Heart Jarvik 2000 MicroMed DeBakey	HVAD DuraHeart HeartMate 3

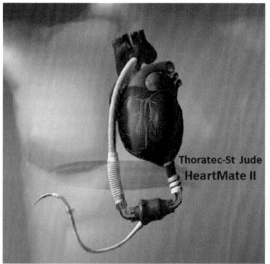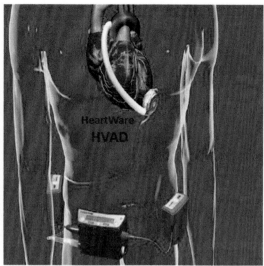

Thoratec-St Jude
HeartMate II

HeartWare
HVAD

Fig. 1. Typical configuration of LVAD support. The LVAD inflow cannula is inserted within the LV apex. Blood is delivered through a motor into the ascending aorta via an outflow graft. Power is supplied externally by batteries worn in harnesses on the patient. (*Courtesy of* St. Jude/Thoratec, Pleasanton, CA, with permission; and HeartWare, Framingham, MA, with permission.)

transplant listing. Other seemingly perfect BTT patients can develop devastating complications after VAD or allosensitization that make finding a donor organ impossible. In a study of 2816 LVAD patients enrolled into INTERMACS, 43.5% of 1060 patients who were listed for cardiac transplant at the time of MCS implant were no longer listed for transplant (ie, converted to DT) at 2 years. In the subset of patients deemed possibly eligible for transplant but not listed (also known as bridge to candidacy, n = 1162) at the time of LVAD implant, 29.3% of these DT patients were eventually transplant listed.[7]

The Centers for Medicare and Medicaid Services–approved criteria for LVAD implant for DT or as a BTT are shown in **Box 1**.[8] Selected contraindications for device support are shown in **Box 2**. The International Society for Heart and Lung Transplant has published guidelines on MCS support inclusion and exclusion criteria to which readers are referred for further detail.[9]

SURVIVAL AFTER LEFT VENTRICULAR ASSIST DEVICES

Outcomes after LVAD implant have made extraordinary gains in the past decade. The HeartMate XVE (St. Jude Medical-Thoratec, Little Canada, Minnesota) was the first FDA-approved device for support in transplant-ineligible patients. In the landmark REMATCH (Randomized Evaluation of Mechanical Assistance for the Treatment of Congestive Heart Failure) trial, 129 patients with end-stage systolic (LV ejection fraction <25%) HF and NYHA class IV symptoms (72% on

inotropes) were randomized to either HeartMate XVE LVAD therapy or to continued medical management.[10] Survival at 1 year was 52% in XVE-supported patients compared with a dismal 25%

Box 1
Centers for Medicare and Medicaid Services–approved indications for LVAD support

DT: FDA approved only for patients with NYHA class IV HF who are not candidates for heart transplant and

1. Patients who have failed optimal medical therapy for at least 45 of the last 60 days or have been balloon pump dependent for 7 days or intravenous inotrope dependent for 14 days

2. LV ejection fraction less than 25%

3. Peak oxygen consumption of $\leq$14 mL/kg/min or unable to perform test

BTT

1. Use of an FDA-approved device implanted according to FDA approval criteria, including NYHA class IV HF

2. Listed for transplant at the time of VAD implant

Data from Centers for Medicare & Medicaid Services. Decision memo for ventricular assist devices as destination therapy (CAG-00119N). Available at: https://www.cms.gov/medicare-coverage-database/details/nca-decision-memo.aspx?NCAId=79&NCDId=4246&ncdver=6&IsPopup=y&bc=AAAAAAAAAgEAAA%3D%3D&. Accessed January 13, 2016.

in the medical therapy group, and gains were noted in measures of quality of life and NYHA functional class after XVE LVAD therapy.[10] An unacceptably high rate of device infection or malfunction requiring LVAD exchange (up to 65% by 2 years of support), however, limited widespread acceptance of the first-generation, pulsatile LVADs.[11] In addition, the XVE device was large, limiting its use in women, adolescents, and anyone else with a body surface area less than or equal to 1.5 m^2.

With technological innovation, second-generation and third-generation CF technologies subsequently emerged. The HeartMate II (HMII) (St. Jude Medical-Thoratec) was the first FDA-approved axial-flow CF-LVAD, obtaining the BTT indication in 2008 and DT approval in 2010.[12,13] Subsequently, the HVAD (HeartWare, Framingham, MA), a petite centrifugally driven, partial magnetic-levitation CF-LVAD, was FDA approved in 2012 for BTT support.[14] The advancements in technology along with improvements in patient selection and device management imparted marked improvements in patient morbidity and mortality. In just 10 years, 1-year survival improved from 52% with first-generation support devices to 80% to 85% for patients on CF support,[3,10–17] with greatest survival gains consistently noted in those supported for the BTT indication. **Fig. 2** and **Table 2** summarize survival statistics from major trials or registries of LVAD support.

SECONDARY BENEFITS OF LEFT VENTRICULAR ASSIST DEVICE SUPPORT

In addition to gains in survival, MCS has fostered marked improvements in other critical facets of patient health. Patient 6-minute walk distances increase an average of 129 m to 185 m[14,16–18] from baseline after LVAD support, and marked improvements in NYHA functional class are enjoyed, with approximately 80% to 83% of patients describing NYHA class I/II symptoms (from class IV at implant) by 18 to 24 months[13,16,17] postoperatively. Quality-of-life measures, including the Kansas City Cardiomyopathy Questionnaire and the EuroQol-5D visual analogue scale, also consistently improve after LVAD support[14–16,18] and such improvements are maintained out to 2 years.[3] Finally, with improved cardiac output on LVAD support, patients typically demonstrate improvements in renal function, hepatic function, and nutritional status.[19–21]

COMPLICATIONS

Despite the marked improvements (discussed previously) in short-term patient survival,

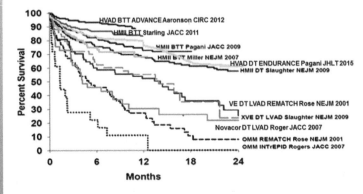

Fig. 2. Survival curves of major clinical trials and registries of LVAD support. (Adapted from Jorde UP, Kushwaha SS, Tatooles AJ, et al. Results of the destination therapy post-Food and Drug Administration approval study with a continuous flow left ventricular assist device: a prospective study using the INTERMACS registry (Interagency Registry for Mechanically Assisted Circulatory Support). J Am Coll Cardiol 2014; 63(21):1756; with permission.)

Table 2
Survival after left ventricular assist device in major clinical trials and INTERMACS

Trial	Device(s) Studied, n	Survival		
		Operative (%)	6 mo (%)	1 y (%)
REMATCH[10]	68 XVE	88	61	52
	61 OMM	—	52	25
HMII-DT[13]	134 HMII	93	78	68
	66 XVE	89	64	55
HMII-BTT[12]	133	89	75	68
HMII-BTT Pivotal[17]	281	92	82	73
INTERMACS-HMII BTT[15]	169	96	91	85
ADVANCE-HeartWare BTT[14]	140 HVAD	99	94	86
	499 HMII	97	92	85
INTERMACS[3]	12,030 CF-LVADs	95	85	80

Abbreviation: OMM, optimal medical management.

long-term survival on MCS support averages approximately 50% at 3.7 years.[3] Although device failure with CF-LVAD support is rare, complications attributable to device support are common. Freedom from major adverse events is only 30% and 14% at 12 months and 36 months, respectively, after VAD implant.[22] The burden of individual adverse events is presented in **Table 3** and a bulleted summary of key complications is presented later. Interpretation of these complications should also include an appreciation of the variable metrics used to describe the events (eg, events per year and events per patient-year [EPPY]).

Bleeding

Bleeding is the most common complication after LVAD implantation. In the HMII BTT trial, the

Table 3
Rates of major events after left ventricular assist implant (2012–2014) based on INTERMACS

Event	n Events (n = 7286)	Rate (Events Per Patient-Year)
Bleeding	4420	7.79
RVF	276	0.49
Infection	4132	7.28
Stroke	916	1.61
Renal dysfunction	876	1.54
Respiratory failure	1551	2.73
Hemolysis	314	0.55

Data from Kirklin JK, Naftel DC, Pagani FD. Seventh INTERMACS annual report: a 15,000 patients and counting. J Heart Lung Transplant 2015;34:1495–504.

frequency of bleeding requiring reoperation was 31%, and 53% of patients received at least 2 units of red blood cells in the postoperative period.[12] Management of bleeding in LVAD patients can be complicated given increased risks for device thrombosis when anticoagulation and antiplatelet therapies are interrupted.[23] VAD centers have individual protocols in place for anticoagulation management during bleeding events. In general, INR reversal is rarely undertaken except in cases of severe exsanguination, large intracranial hemorrhage, or need for emergent surgery.

- Causes of early postoperative bleeding include diffuse coagulopathy in the setting of hepatic congestion or ischemia, hemodilution of clotting factors during bypass, consumption of clotting factors during surgery, and residual effects of antiplatelet therapies used preoperatively.[24]
- Causes of later bleeding include the need for chronic antiplatelet and anticoagulant therapy, the development of arteriovenous malformations,[25–27] hepatic dysfunction from postimplant right ventricular failure (RVF), and acquired von Willebrand syndrome.

Approximately 100% of patients after CF-LVAD implant have deficiencies in von Willebrand high-molecular-weight multimers, presumably due to rheologic trauma to these large proteins. This bleeding tendency is also exacerbated by the related formation of arteriovenous malformations in the gastrointestinal tract (20%–44% gastrointestinal bleed incidence after VAD), spleen (spontaneous splenic rupture), lung (pulmonary hemorrhage), nasopharynx (recurrent epistaxis), and brain (intracranial hemorrhage).[23,25–28]

Stroke

Patients on CF-LVAD support have increased risk for hemorrhagic and ischemic stroke.

- In INTERMACS (n = 5300 patients with CF-LVAD), freedom from stroke rates were 89% and 83% at 1 and 2 years, respectively.[22]
- There is a suggestion of increased stroke risk during HVAD compared with HMII support. In the HMII BTT trial, event rates for ischemic and hemorrhagic stroke were 0.04 EPPY and 0.05 EPPY,[29] respectively, compared with rates of 0.11 EPPY and 0.09 EPPY, respectively, in the HeartWare ADVANCE (Evaluation of the HeartWare Left Ventricular Assist Device for the Treatment of Advanced Heart Failure) BTT trial.[14] The ENDURANCE trial compared outcomes in HMII- and HVAD-supported DT patients.[16] Ischemic stroke rates were 0.06 EPPY and 0.16 EPPY for the HMII versus HVAD, respectively ($P = .02$), and hemorrhagic stroke rates were 0.03 EPPY and 0.11 EPPY, respectively ($P = .001$).[16]
- Risk factors for thromboembolic events on MCS include type 2 diabetes mellitus, female gender,[28] older age,[29] low INR, device thrombosis/hemolysis,[30] and higher mean arterial pressure.[16]

Infection

The presence of an external driveline with direct communication to the environment exposes patients to a constant hazard for infection. Although infection often starts locally at the driveline exit site, organisms can quickly extend to the pump or spread hematogenously elsewhere.

- The rate of major infection in the present era of MCS is 7.3 EPPY.[3]
- Obesity, younger age, diabetes, protein calorie malnutrition, and driveline trauma are a few risk factors for systemic and driveline infections.[31–34]
- Most infections are caused by skin organisms (*Staphylococcus* and *Streptococcus*). *Pseudomonas* and methicillin-resistant *Staphylococcal aureus* infections seem to confer the highest morbidity and mortality.[34,35]
- The best means of reducing the morbidity and mortality associated with a device infection is prevention. Centers have individualized preoperative and postoperative antibiotic prophylaxis regimens. Driveline care includes frequent sterile dressing changes and use of a driveline restraint device to minimize driveline movement.
- For patients who have recurrent driveline infections or fail to clear cultures with concern

for pump infection, device exchange and cardiac transplant (if eligible) are the recommended interventions. Studies consistently show increased morbidity (including increased risks of device thrombosis and stroke) and mortality after driveline infection and rates of sepsis are 17% to 26%, respectively.[31–35]
- Consideration for infection of the VAD and/or its other component parts should always be had, especially when there are positive blood cultures, cryptic fevers, failure to resolve an infectious clinical picture with antibiotics, and/or recurrent embolic events. Device exchange or cardiac transplant is required for cure.

Device Thrombosis

Baseline frequencies of device thrombosis in INTERMACS and clinical trials were initially reported at 2% to 3% at 1 year postimplant but there was a rise in reported LVAD thrombosis rates to 6% to 7% beginning in the years 2011 to 2012.[14–16,36,37] The increased rates were exclusive to the HMII device. Reasons for the uptrend in device thrombosis remain unclear but are likely multifactorial, including changes in intensity of anticoagulation regimens, variable monitoring of thrombosis laboratories, and better diagnosis/awareness of device thrombosis by MCS practitioners.

- VAD thrombosis is associated with increased mortality and morbidity, including increased risks for stroke (hazard ratio 3.6) and need for device exchange.[30,36] Survival after device exchange for thrombosis is poor: 59% at 2 years compared with 69% after primary device implant.[36] In 1 series, mortality after pump thrombosis in those without device exchange was 48% 6 months.[37]
- Diagnosis of VAD thrombosis requires a careful clinical history and multimodality testing approach. Clinical symptoms include hemoglobinuria (tea-colored urine) and recurrent HF symptoms. Laboratory abnormalities include an elevated lactate dehydrogenase and serum-free hemoglobin and reduced haptoglobin and hemoglobin—all markers of red blood cell destruction from hemolysis induced by turbulent flow through a CF-LVAD. Of these markers, an elevated lactate dehydrogenase greater than 2.5 times the upper limit of laboratory normal offers the highest sensitivity and specificity for detecting device thrombosis.[30,38]
- Elevated device power consumption can be a sign of device thrombosis but power

elevations are a low-sensitivity[30] tool for thrombosis detection.

- Echocardiography can demonstrate poor LVAD unloading of the left ventricle manifested as a failure to close the aortic valve and failure to reduce LV dimensions despite sequential increases in pump speed (known as a ramp protocol).[39]

Right Ventricular Railure

RVF can occur acutely after LVAD implant or can be a slowly progressive complication with onset months after LVAD implant. Defining the incidence of RVF after VAD is complicated by lack of a consistent definition used in clinical study but rates in INTERAMCS are 0.49 EPPY.

- Definitions for RVF by MCS investigators have included the intraoperative or postoperative use of surgical or temporary RVAD support, prolonged (eg, 7–14 days) use of postoperative inotropes or pulmonary vasodilators, and/or elevated central venous pressures with a reduced cardiac index.
- RVF can occur acutely after LVAD implant due to increased preload delivered from the LVAD or from adverse shift of the interventricular septum away from the right ventricle (RV) in the setting of aggressive LVAD speed settings. Exacerbation of pulmonary hypertension due to perioperative blood product transfusions, hypoxia, or acidosis can also increase RV wall stress and induce RVF. Published acute RVF incidences vary from 15% to 35%.[13,14,16,18,40]
- In the preoperative setting, a careful assessment of RV function is critical. Right heart catheterization and echocardiography are obligatory. Use of pulmonary vasodilators (including nitrates and milrinone) and aggressive volume management to reduce preoperative right atrial pressure and wedge pressure are recommended.
- Several risk predictors for post-LVAD acute RVF exist but accuracy remains poor given the multifactorial nature RVF development. Correlates of risk include need for vasopressor support; elevated creatinine, bilirubin, aspartate aminotransferase, and/or INR; female gender; markers of RV dysfunction by echocardiography (lower tricuspid annular plane systolic excursion, lower strain rates, smaller LV internal dimension, and larger RV:LV internal dimension ratio); and right heart catheterization (RV stroke work index, pulmonary artery pulsatility index).[40–46]

ENSURING GOOD OUTCOMES FOR LEFT VENTRICULAR ASSIST DEVICE–SUPPORTED PATIENTS

Early referral and careful patient selection are obligatory to achieving good patient outcomes after LVAD implant. Patient referral to an advanced HF specialist prior to the onset of organ failure and cachexia (eg, NYHA class III) allows for preparation/education of a patient about prognosis and treatment options, including LVAD support, development of family/patient trust in the MCS practitioner, and a planned approach to LVAD implant when deemed necessary.

- Several inpatient and outpatient studies have identified markers of increased risk of death from medical management of systolic HF. In general, frequent admission for HF management (>1 in 6 months), inability to tolerate doses of evidence-based HF medications due to hypotension, worsening renal function, escalating diuretics and/or use of a primer (sequential nephron blockade), and recurrent ventricular dysrhythmias are high-risk signs.[47–49]
- After identification of high-risk HF patients, the MCS practitioner must determine if the patient can survive the MCS operative intervention with acceptable morbidity and mortality. Several risk scores have been devised to predict operative risk and select scores are summarized in **Table 4**.[50–55]
- The HMII risk score (HMRS) is a risk prediction tool to assist in risk stratification of patients being considered for CF-LVAD support.[50,54] The original HMRS formula is with low-risk (HMRS <1.58), medium-risk (1.58–2.48), and high-risk (HMRS >2.48) groups for predicting 90-day mortality after HMII LVAD implant[50]:

HMRS = $(0.0274 \times [\text{age in years}]) - (0.723 \times [\text{albumin g/dL}]) + (0.74 \times [\text{creatinine mg/dL}]) + (1.136 \times [\text{INR}]) + (0.807 \times [\text{center volume} >15])$ (A value of 1.0 is entered for LVAD center volume <15)

- An adjusted HMRS omits center volume (defined previously based on clinical trial volume and not true center LVAD volume) with very low–risk (score <0.20), low-risk (score 0.20–1.97), medium-risk (score 1.98–4.48), and high-risk (score >4.48) score thresholds for 90-day mortality.[54] The adjusted HMRS

Table 4
Summary of select risk scores

Trial	Cohort	Variables in Score Formula				
HMRS[50]	HMII BTT and DT trial patients (n = 1122)	↑ Age	↑ Creatinine	↑ INR	↓ Albumin	↓ Center volume
AdjHMRS[54]	HVAD BTT trial (n = 360) patients and INTERMACS (n = 9773)	↑ Age	↑ Creatinine	↑ INR	↓ Albumin	—
MELD[51]	Single center (n = 211) and INTERMACS (n = 324); largely first-generation devices	↑ Bilirubin	↑ Creatinine	↑ INR		
TVAD[52]	Single center; n = 10 CF-LVAD and n = 49 other	↑ Bilirubin	↑ LV Diastolic dimension	↑ Central venous pressure	↓ Albumin	
Lietz-Miller DT score[53]	HeartMate XVE (n = 280) DT patients	↓ Platelets ↑ AST	Vasodilator use ↓ Hematocrit	↑ INR ↑ Serum urea nitrogen	↓ Albumin No inotrope	↓ Mean pulmonary pressure —
Revised screening scale[55]	HeartMate VE (n = 130)	Preoperative ventilator	Preoperative MCS	↑ PT	↑ Central venous pressure	Postcardiotomy failure

Abbreviations: AdjHMRS, Adjusted HeartMate II Risk Score; HMRS, HeartMate II Risk Score; MELD, Model for End-stage Liver Disease; TVAD, TODAI Ventricular Assist Device.

has validation within INTERMACS and for the HVAD[54]:

$$HMRS \text{ adjusted} = (0.0274 \times [\text{age in years}]) - (0.723 \times [\text{albumin g/dL}]) + (0.74 \times [\text{creatinine mg/dL}]) + (1.136 \times [\text{INR}])$$

- In general, presence of cardiogenic shock, older age, advanced irreversible renal dysfunction (creatinine that fails to improve with improved cardiac output delivered via inotropes and/or a balloon pump or temporary mechanical support), and RVF are high-risk markers for poor outcome after LVAD.[50–55]

SUMMARY

In the past decade, there has been a dramatic evolution in the field of MCS. Device-related complications continue to burden the field and will be a major obstacle for achieving therapeutic noninferiority in comparison with cardiac transplant. Selected patients with end-stage systolic HF, however, now enjoy an average survival of 80% at 1 year post-VAD implant, which is vastly better than survival rates of 25% to 50% on chronic inotrope support. Early patient referral to an advanced HF specialist before the onset of significant end-organ dysfunction and malnutrition is critical for achieving good operative outcomes on LVAD support.

REFERENCES

1. Mozaffarian D, Benjamin EJ, Go AS, et al. Heart disease and stroke statistics- 2015 update. A report from the American Heart Association. Circulation 2016;133:e38–360.
2. Costanzo MR, Mills RM, Wynne J. Characteristics of "stage D" heart failure: insights from the Acute Decompensated Heart Failure National Registry Longitudinal Module (ADHERE LM). Am Heart J 2008;155:339–47.
3. Kirklin JK, Naftel DC, Pagani FD. Seventh INTERMACS annual report: a 15,000 patients and counting. J Heart Lung Transplant 2015;34:1495–504.
4. Joyce DL, Conte JV, Russell SD, et al. Disparities in access to left ventricular assist device therapy. J Surg Res 2009;152:111–7.
5. HeartMate II LVAS patient management guidelines. Available at: http://www.fda.gov/ohrms/dockets/ac/07/briefing/2007-4333b2-20-%209_4%20HM%20II%20Patient%20Management%20Guidelines.pdf. Accessed January 13, 2016.
6. HeartWare ventricular assist system instructions for use. Available at: http://www.heartware.com/sites/default/files/uploads/docs/ifu00001_rev_15.pdf. Accessed January 13, 2016.
7. Teuteberg JJ, Stewart GC, Jessup M, et al. Implant strategies change over time and impact outcomes: insights from the INTERMACS (Interagency Registry for Mechanically Assisted Circulatory Support). JACC Heart Fail 2013;1:369–78.
8. CMS approved indications. Available at: https://www.cms.gov/medicare-coverage-database/details/nca-decision-memo.aspx?NCAId=79&NCDId=246&ncdver=6&IsPopup=y&bc=AAAAAAAAAgEAAA%3D%3D&. Accessed January 13, 2016.
9. Feldman D, Pamboukian SV, Teuteberg J, et al. The 2013 International Society for Heart and Lung Transplantation Guidelines for mechanical circulatory support: executive summary. J Heart Lung Transplant 2013;32:157–87.
10. Rose EA, Gelijns AC, Moskowitz AJ, et al. Long-term use of a left ventricular assist device for end-stage heart failure. The Randomized Evaluation of Mechanical Assistance for the Treatment of Congestive Heart Failure (REMATCH) Study Group. N Engl J Med 2001;345:1435–43.
11. Dembitsky WP, Tector AJ, Park S, et al. Left ventricular assist device performance with long-term circulatory support: lessons from the REMATCH trial. Ann Thorac Surg 2004;78:2123–9.
12. Miller LW, Pagani FD, Russell SD, et al. Use of a continuous flow device in patients awaiting heart transplantation. N Engl J Med 2007;357:885–96.
13. Slaughter MS, Roger JG, Milan CA, et al. Advanced heart failure treated with a continuous flow left ventricular assist device. N Engl J Med 2009;361:2241–51.
14. Aaronson KD, Slaughter MS, Miller LW, et al. Use of an intrapericardial continuous flow centrifugal pump in patients awaiting heart transplantation. Circulation 2012;125:3191–200.
15. Starling RC, Naka Y, Boyle AJ, et al. Results of the post-US Food and Drug Administration-Approval study with a continuous flow left ventricular assist device as a bridge to heart transplantation. J Am Coll Cardiol 2011;57:1890–8.
16. Pagani FD, Milano CM, Tatooles AJ, et al. HeartWare HVAD for the treatment of patients with advanced heart failure ineligible for cardiac transplantation: results of the ENDURANCE destination therapy trial. J Heart Lung Transplant 2015;34:S9.
17. Pagani FD, Miller LW, Russell SD, et al. Extended mechanical circulatory support with a continuous flow rotary left ventricular assist device. J Am Coll Cardiol 2009;54:312–21.
18. Slaughter MS, Pagani FD, McGee EC, et al. Heartware ventricular assist system for bridge to transplant: combined results of the bridge to transplant and continued access protocol trial. The HeartWare Bridge to transplant ADVANCE trial. J Heart Lung Transplant 2013;32:675–83.

19. Demirozu ZT, Etheridge WB, Radovancevic R, et al. Results of HeartMate II left ventricular assist device implantation on renal function in patients requiring post-implant renal replacement therapy. J Heart Lung Transplant 2011;30:182–7.

20. Deo SV, Sharma V, Altarabsheh SE, et al. Hepatic and renal function with successful long-term support on a continuous flow left ventricular assist device. Heart Lung Circ 2014;23:229–33.

21. Hasin T, Topilsky Y, Schirger JA, et al. Changes in renal function after implantation of continuous-flow left ventricular assist devices. J Am Coll Cardiol 2012;59:26–36.

22. Kirklin JK, Naftel DC, Kormos RL, et al. Fifth INTER-MACS annual report: risk factor analysis from more than 6,000 mechanical circulatory support patients. J Heart Lung Transplant 2013;32:141–56.

23. Stulak JM, Lee D, Haft JW, et al. Gastrointestinal bleeding and subsequent risk of thromboembolic events during support with a left ventricular assist device. J Heart Lung Transplant 2014;33:60–4.

24. Despotis GJ, Avidan MS, Hoque CW. Mechanisms and attenuation of hemostatic activation during extracorporeal circulation. Ann Thorac Surg 2001; 72:S1821–31.

25. Suarez J, Patel CB, Felker GM, et al. Mechanisms of bleeding and approach to patients with axial-flow left ventricular assist devices. Circ Heart Fail 2011; 4:779–84.

26. Uriel N, Pak SW, Jorde UP, et al. Acquired von Willebrand syndrome after continuous flow mechanical device support contributes to a high prevalence of bleeding during long term support and at the time of transplantation. J Am Coll Cardiol 2010;56: 1207–13.

27. Draper KV, Huang RJ, Gerson LB. GI Bleeding in patients with continuous flow left ventricular assist devices: a systemic review and metanalysis. Gastrointest Endosc 2014;80:435–46.

28. Boyle AJ, Jorde UP, Sun B, et al. Preoperative risk factors of bleeding and stroke during left ventricular assist device support. An analysis of more than 900 HeartMate II outpatients. J Am Coll Cardiol 2014;63: 880–8.

29. Coffin ST, Haglund NA, Davis ME, et al. Adverse neurologic events in patients bridged with long-term mechanical circulatory support: a device-specific comparative analysis. J Heart Lung Transplant 2015;34:1578–85.

30. Cowger JA, Romano MA, Shah P, et al. Hemolysis: a harbinger of adverse outcome after left ventricular assist device implant. J Heart Lung Transplant 2014;33:35–43.

31. John R, Aaronson KD, Pae WE, et al. Driveline infections and sepsis in patients receiving the HVAD system as a left ventricular assist device. J Heart Lung Transplant 2014;33:1066–73.

32. Goldstein DJ, Naftel D, Holman W, et al. Continuous flow devices and percutaneous site infections: clinical outcomes. J Heart Lung Transplant 2012;31: 1151–7.

33. Trachtenberg BH, Cordero-Reyes AM, Aldeiri M, et al. Persistent blood stream infection in patients supported with a continuous-flow left ventricular assist device is associated with an increased risk of cerebrovascular accidents. J Card Fail 2015; 21(2):119–25.

34. Koval CE, Thuita L, Moazami N, et al. Evolution and impact of drive-line infection in a large cohort of continuous flow ventricular assist device recipients. J Heart Lung Transplant 2014;33:1164–72.

35. Topkara VK, Kondareddy S, Malik F, et al. Infectious complications in patients with left ventricular assist device: etiology and outcomes in the continuous-flow era. Ann Thorac Surg 2010;90(4):1270–7.

36. Kirklin JK, Naftel DC, Kormos RL, et al. Interagency Registry for Mechanically Assisted Circulatory Support (INTERMACS) analysis of pump thrombosis in the HeartMate II left ventricular assist device. J Heart Lung Transplant 2014;33:12–22.

37. Starling RC, Moazami N, Silvestry SC. Unexpected abrupt increase in left ventricular assist device thrombosis. N Engl J Med 2014;370:33–40.

38. Shah P, Mehta VM, Cowger JA, et al. Diagnosis of hemolysis and device thrombosis with lactate dehydrogenase during left ventricular assist device support. J Heart Lung Transplant 2014;33:102–4.

39. Uriel N, Morrison KA, Garan AR, et al. Development of a novel echocardiography ramp test for speed optimization and diagnosis of device thrombosis in continuous-flow left ventricular assist devices: the Columbia ramp study. J Am Coll Cardiol 2012;60: 1764–75.

40. Matthews JC, Koelling TM, Pagani FD, et al. The right ventricular failure risk score a pre-operative tool for assessing the risk of right ventricular failure in left ventricular assist device candidates. J Am Coll Cardiol 2008;51:2163–72.

41. Fitzpatrick JF, Frederick JR, Hsu VM, et al. Risk score derived from preoperative data analysis predicts the need for biventricular mechanical support. J Heart Lung Transplant 2008;27:1286–92.

42. Ochiai Y, McCarthy PM, Smedira NG, et al. Predictors of severe right ventricular failure after implantable left ventricular assist system insertion: analysis of 245 patients. Circulation 2002;106: I198–202.

43. Lampert BC, Teuteberg JJ. Right ventricular failure after left ventricular assist devices. J Heart Lung Transplant 2015;34:1123–30.

44. Neyer J, Arsanjani R, Moriguchi J, et al. Echocardiographic parameters associated with right ventricular failure after left ventricular assist device: a review. J Heart Lung Transplant 2016;35(3):283–93.

45. Kang G, Ha R, Banerjee D. Pulmonary artery pulsatility index predicts right ventricular failure after left ventricular assist device implantation. J Heart Lung Transplant 2016;35:67–73.

46. Kalogeropoulos AP, Kelka A, Weinberger JF. Validation of clinical scores for right ventricular failure prediction after implantation of continuous flow left ventricular assist devices. J Heart Lung Transplant 2015;34:1595–603.

47. Levy WC, Mozaffarian D, Linker DT, et al. The seattle heart failure model: prediction of survival in heart failure. Circulation 2006;113:1424–33.

48. Fleming LM, Gavin M, Piatkowski G, et al. Derivation and validation of a 30 day heart failure readmission model. Am J Cardiol 2014;114:1379–82.

49. Rahimi K, Bennett D, Conrad N, et al. Risk prediction in patients with heart failure: a systematic review and analysis. JACC Heart Fail 2014;2:440–6.

50. Cowger JA, Sundareswaran K, Rogers JG, et al. Predicting survival in patients receiving continuous flow left ventricular assist devices: the HeartMate II risk score. J Am Coll Cardiol 2013;61:313–21.

51. Matthews JC, Pagani FD, Haft JW, et al. Model for end stage liver disease score predicts left ventricular assist device operative transfusion requirements, morbidity, and mortality. Circulation 2010;121:214–20.

52. Imamura T, Kinugawa K, Shiga T, et al. Novel risk scoring system with preoperative objective parameters gives a good prediction of 1-year mortality in patients with a left ventricular assist device. Circ J 2012;76:1895–903.

53. Lietz K, Long JW, Kfoury AG, et al. Outcomes of left ventricular assist device implantation as destination therapy in the post-REMATCH era: implications for patient selection. Circulation 2007;116:497–505.

54. Cowger JA, Castle L, Aaronson KD, et al. The HeartMate II risk score: an adjusted score for evaluation of all continuous flow left ventricular assist devices. ASAIO J 2016. [Epub ahead of print].

55. Rao V, Oz MC, Flannery MA, et al. Revised Screening scale to predict survival after insertion of a left ventricular assist device. J Thorac Cardiovasc Surg 2003;125:855–62.

Changing Role of Heart Transplantation

Michelle M. Kittleson, MD, PhD

KEYWORDS

- Heart transplantation • Heart transplant allocation • Primary graft dysfunction • Sensitization
- Rituximab • Bortezomib • Eculizumab

KEY POINTS

- Proposed changes to the heart transplant allocation policy may reduce waitlist mortality for the most critically ill candidates without a detrimental effect on posttransplant survival.
- Primary graft dysfunction is likely to increase as heart transplants are performed in older recipients with more comorbidities using older donors
- Advances to shorten ischemic time with an ex vivo perfusion platform may mitigate this risk.
- Identification of potentially cytotoxic donor-specific anti-HLA antibodies before transplantation offers hope of heart transplantation for highly sensitized candidates.

INTRODUCTION

Despite advances in pharmacologic and device treatment of chronic heart failure, long-term morbidity and mortality remain high and many patients progress to end-stage heart failure. The 5-year mortality for patients with symptomatic heart failure approaches 50%, and may be as high as 80% at 1 year for end-stage patients.[1–3] Over the last 4 decades, cardiac transplantation has become the preferred therapy for select patients with end-stage heart disease, with a 1-year survival post heart transplantation of almost 90% and a conditional half-life of 13 years (**Fig. 1**),[4] certainly far better than one could expect from end-stage heart failure.

Although heart transplantation has become standard of care for the management of end-stage heart failure, the role of heart transplantation in the United States is changing as the characteristics of heart transplant candidates continue to evolve. The number of patients with end-stage heart failure is increasing, and the number of donor organs remains constant and a limiting factor in transplantation.[5] Not only are there more potential heart transplant candidates, but heart transplant candidates today more complex. The proportion of candidates aged 65 years or older has increased: in 2013, 18.2% of candidates were aged 65 years or older, compared with 10.8% in 2003.[5] The proportion of candidates with mechanical circulatory support (most commonly ventricular assist devices [VADs]) at listing has also increased dramatically, from 7.5% in 2003% to 27.4% in 2013[5] and the proportion of patients transplanted from VADs has increased as well[4] (**Fig. 2**). Furthermore, the number of heart transplant candidates with antibodies to HLA, so-called sensitization is increasing over the past decade.[6]

Thus, the heart transplant candidates of the modern era are older, sensitized, with mechanical circulatory support, and at higher risk for poor outcomes, including primary graft dysfunction (PGD) and antibody-mediated rejection.[4,5,7] This article focuses on recent advances in heart transplantation that could address these challenges. These developments include (1) proposed changes in heart transplant allocation policy for more

Disclosures: None.

Division of Cardiology, Cedars-Sinai Heart Institute, 8536 Wilshire Boulevard, Suite 301, Los Angeles, CA 90211, USA

E-mail address: michelle.kittleson@cshs.org

Heart Failure Clin 12 (2016) 411–421

http://dx.doi.org/10.1016/j.hfc.2016.03.004

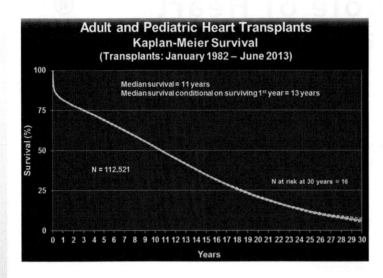

Fig. 1. Survival after heart transplantation. Actuarial survival for adult and pediatric heart transplants patients performed between January 1982 and June 2013. The half-life is the time at which 50% of those transplanted remain alive, and the conditional half-life is the time to 50% survival for recipients surviving the first year after transplantation. (*Data from* Lund LH, Edwards LB, Kucheryavaya AY, et al. The registry of the international society for heart and lung transplantation: thirty-second official adult heart transplantation report—2015; focus theme: early graft failure. J Heart Lung Transplant 2015;34(10):1249.)

equitable organ distribution, (2) a better understanding of the definition and management of PGD, and (3) advances in the management of sensitized heart transplant candidates. Developments in these areas could result in more equitable distribution and expansion of the donor pool and improved quality of life and survival for heart transplant recipients.

HEART TRANSPLANT ALLOCATION POLICY
Current System

Allocation of thoracic organs in the United States is made according to the recipient's priority on the United Network for Organ Sharing waiting list and geographic distance from the donor. Priority on the recipient waiting list is determined by a recipient's assigned status code and time accrued within a status code. In general, patients with the highest medical urgency and lowest expected short-term survival are assigned a higher status code.[8] Donor hearts are first offered to local status 1 patients and then extended to status 1 patients within a 500-mile radius of the donor hospital (zone A). If no eligible recipients are identified, the organ is offered to local status 2 patients. This process repeats in a sequence of "zones" delineated by subsequent concentric circles of 1000- and 1500-mile radii from the donor hospital.

In the current system, there is marked regional variability in waitlist time.[9] As shown in **Fig. 3**, the median wait time for status 1A patients between 2006 and 2012 ranges from a low of 8 days in region 8, comprising the Great Plains states, to a high of 50 days in region 1, which includes the Northeastern states. Options to increase regional access to potential donors include offering hearts to status 1A candidates across a broader

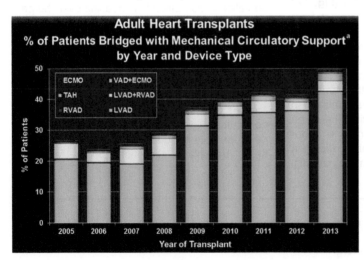

Fig. 2. Mechanical circulatory support as bridge to transplant. Use of mechanical circulatory support to bridge patients to transplant, predominantly in the form of left VAD (LVAD), is increasing over time with 42% transplanted from LVADs in 2013, and there was a resurgence in use of extracorporeal membrane oxygenation (ECMO), reaching 0.9% in 2013. RVAD, right VAD; TAH, total artificial heart. [a] LVAD, RVAD, TAH, ECMO. (*From* Lund LH, Edwards LB, Kucheryavaya AY, et al. The registry of the international society for heart and lung transplantation: thirty-second official adult heart transplantation report—2015; focus theme: early graft failure. J Heart Lung Transplant 2015; 34(10):1249; with permission.)

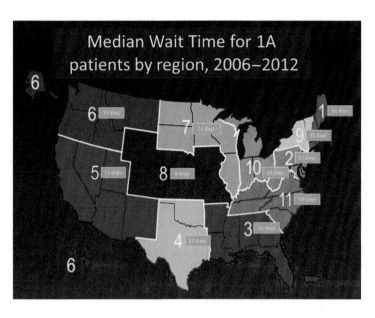

Fig. 3. Regional wait time variation. The median wait time for status 1A patients by United Network for Organ Sharing region illustrates the significant regional variation. (*Data from* Schulze PC, Kitada S, Clerkin K, et al. Regional differences in recipient waitlist time and pre- and post-transplant mortality after the 2006 united network for organ sharing policy changes in the donor heart allocation algorithm. JACC Heart Fail 2014;2(2):166–77.)

geographic area before allocating the hearts to status 1B and 2 candidates as well as eliminating local zone allocation altogether. Modeling geographic heart allocation is expected to occur after the completion of the overall tiered allocation structure described elsewhere in this paper.

The Need for a New Approach

This process is seemingly equitable in that the sickest patients who have been waiting the longest will be considered first when a donor heart becomes available. However, changes in the heart transplant landscape have motivated efforts to improve the current system[10–12] (**Box 1**). The goals of the revision are to increase transplantation rates for adult candidates with the highest waiting list mortality rates and to achieve the greatest survival benefit for heart transplant recipients.

Box 1
Motivation to change the current system of heart transplant allocation

- There is an increase in candidates awaiting transplantation without a corresponding increase in donors.

- The highest acuity (status 1A) patients have undesirably high mortality.

- Advances in durable mechanical support have improved mortality in this subset of the waiting list.

- There is increasing geographical variability in waiting list times.

The current status criteria are shown in **Table 1**. There are 2 major problems with the current criteria. First, the system offers inadequate resolution. For example, status 1A includes patients supported with extracorporeal membrane oxygenation, mechanical ventilation, and inotropic support and continuous hemodynamic monitoring, and all have equal urgency. However, heart transplant candidates on extracorporeal membrane oxygenation support are more tenuous with lower projected survival than candidates receiving low-dose support from 2 inotropic agents and continuous hemodynamic monitoring; yet 2 such patients would receive the same priority under the current 3-tiered system. Second, the current system ignores candidates with a poor prognosis who would not qualify for traditional status 1A listing with inotropic support and continuous hemodynamic monitoring, such as those with complex congenital heart disease, restrictive or infiltrative cardiomyopathies, or refractory ventricular tachycardia.[10,11]

Changing the Heart Allocation Policy

Proposed changes to this system focus on moving from the current 3-tiered system to a multiple-tiered system that better captures the medical urgency of the highest acuity patients (**Table 2**). This multiple-tiered system prioritizes patients supported with extracorporeal membrane oxygenation, mechanical ventilation, nondischargeable VADs, and mechanical circulatory support with life-threatening arrhythmias in the highest tier above those patients with uncomplicated

Table 1
Current status codes for heart transplant allocation

Status Code	Criteria
Status 1A	• ECMO • IABP • Inpatient TAH • Mechanical ventilation • Continuous infusion of a single high-dose intravenous inotrope or multiple intravenous inotropes, and with continuous hemodynamic monitoring of left ventricular filling pressures • LVAD, RVAD, or BiVAD for 30 d • Mechanical circulatory support with significant device-related complications (thromboembolism, device infection, mechanical failure, or life-threatening ventricular arrhythmias).
Status 1B	• Uncomplicated LVAD, RVAD, BiVAD after 30 d have been used • Outpatient TAH • Continuous infusion of intravenous inotropes
Status 2	Candidates not meeting 1A or 1B criteria
Status 7	Temporarily inactive, most often owing to infection

Abbreviations: BiVAD, biventricular assist device; ECMO, extracorporeal membrane oxygenation; IABP, intraaortic balloon pump; LVAD, left ventricular assist device; RVAD, right ventricular assist device; TAH, total artificial heart.
Data from Organ procurement and transplantation network policy 6.1. Available at: https://optn.transplant.hrsa.gov/media/1200/optn_policies.pdf#nameddest=Policy_06. Accessed March 8, 2016.

mechanical circulatory support or continuous inotropic support with continuous hemodynamic monitoring. The proposed system also addresses potentially underserved populations, such as adults with congenital heart disease, retransplantation, restrictive cardiomyopathy, and hypertrophic cardiomyopathy in a separate tier above current status 2 patients.

A simulation of this proposed system will be performed to determine if waitlist mortality can be decreased while maintaining current levels of posttransplant survival. These efforts should lead to a revision to the current heart transplant allocation scheme that allows for more equitable distribution of the scarce resource of donor organs such that the most critically ill patients are most likely to receive transplantation before the window of viability closes.

PRIMARY GRAFT DYSFUNCTION
Defining Primary Graft Dysfunction

In 2013, a consensus conference, convened to formulate guidelines regarding PGD after heart transplantation, highlighted the significant burden of this problem.[13] In an international survey of 47 heart transplant centers comprising almost 10,000 patients, a PGD rate of 7.4% was reported with a 30-day mortality of 30%. At this conference, a strict definition of PGD was created (**Table 3**). The advantages of a strict definition of PGD include (1) the ability to create future registries to follow the care and outcomes of patients with PGD and (2) an assurance that future studies undertaken to determine risk factors or effect of therapies will include that patients of comparable degree of PGD.

Risk Factors

Part of the changing landscape of transplantation is the increasing age of donors and recipients[4] and the increased acuity of patients awaiting heart transplantation. This translates into an increased risk of PGD, as noted with the RADIAL score, an acronym for a validated risk model for the development of PGD which includes recipient characteristics of Right atrial pressure of greater than10 mm Hg, Age greater than 60 years, Diabetes, Inotrope dependence and donor characteristics of Age greater than 30 years and Length of ischemic time greater than 240 minutes (**Box 2**). Each of the 6 risk factors in the RADIAL score is assigned 1 point with an incidence of PGD of 12%, 19% and 28% for patients with scores of 0 to 1, 2, and 3 or more points, respectively.[14,15]

Management and Potential Prevention

There are no biomarkers for PGD and treatment is supportive (**Fig. 4**). In addition, many of the risk factors for PGD noted in the RADIAL score are not modifiable, such as recipient age, recipient history of diabetes, recipient need for inotropic support, and donor age. However, the length of cold ischemic time could be improved with an ex vivo heart perfusion platform that maintains the donor heart in a warm, beating state for transplantation. In a trial to assess the safety of an ex vivo platform, 130 patients were randomized to receive donor hearts preserved with either the Organ Care System or standard cold storage. There was no difference in 30-day patient and graft survival rates or serious adverse events.[16] An ongoing phase III clinical trial, the International Trial to Evaluate the Safety and Effectiveness of the Portable Organ Care System (OCS) Heart for

Table 2
Proposed new tiers for heart allocation model

Proposed New Tiers	Corresponding Current Tiers
1.	
i. ECMO	Status 1A
ii. Mechanical ventilation	Status 1A
iii. Nondischargeable VAD	Status 1A or 1B
iv. MCS with life-threatening ventricular arrhythmia	Status 1A
2.	
i. IABP	Status 1A
ii. VT/VF without MCS	Status 1A
iii. MCS with device malfunction	Status 1A
iv. TAH	Status 1A or 1B
v. Dischargeable BiVAD or LVAD	Status 1A or 1B
3.	
i. LVAD for up to 30 d	Status 1A
ii. Status 1A exception	Status 1A
iii. Multiple inotropes or single inotrope with continuous hemodynamic monitoring	Status 1A
iv. MCS with device infection	Status 1A
v. MCS with thromboembolism	Status 1A
vi. MCS with other device-related complication not listed above	Status 1A
4.	

i. Diagnosis of CHD with
   a. Unrepaired/incompletely repaired complex CHD, usually with cyanosis
   b. Repaired CHD with 2 ventricles
   c. Single ventricle repairs with Fontan or modifications
	NA

ii. Ischemic heart disease with intractable angina	NA
iii. Hypertrophic cardiomyopathy	NA
iv. Restrictive cardiomyopathy	NA
v. Amyloidosis	NA
vi. Stable LVADs after 30 d	Status 1B
vii. Inotropes without hemodynamic monitoring	Status 1B
viii. Retransplant	NA
ix. Status 1B exceptions	Status 1B
5.	
Approved combined organ transplants: heart-lung, heart-liver, heart-kidney	NA
6.	
All remaining candidates	Status 2
7.	
Inactive/not transplantable candidates	Status 7/inactive

Abbreviations: BiVAD, biventricular assist device; CHD, congenital heart disease; ECMO, extracorporeal membrane oxygenation; IABO, intraaortic balloon pump; LVAD, left ventricular assist device; MCS, mechanical circulatory support; NA, not applicable; TAH, total artificial heart; VAD, ventricular assist device; VT/VF, ventricular tachycardia/ventricular failure.

Adapted from Meyer DM, Rogers JG, Edwards LB, et al. The future direction of the adult heart allocation system in the United States. Am J Transplant 2015;15(1):50; with permission.

Table 3
Definition of severity scale for PGD

PGD-LV	Mild PGD–LV: One of the following criteria must be met	LVEF ≤40% by echocardiography, or hemodynamics with RAP >15 mm Hg, PCWP >20 mm Hg, CI <2.0 L/min/m² (lasting > 1 h) requiring low-dose inotropes
	Moderate PGD-LV: Must meet one criterion from I and another criterion from II:	I. One criterion from the following: Left ventricular ejection fraction <40%, or hemodynamic compromise with RAP >15 mm Hg, PCWP >20 mm Hg, CI <2.0 L/min/m², hypotension with MAP <70 mm Hg (lasting > 1 h) II. One criterion from the following: High-dose inotropes—Inotrope score >10[a] or newly placed IABP (regardless of inotropes)
	Severe PGD–LV	Dependence on left or biventricular mechanical support including ECMO, LVAD, BiVAD, or percutaneous LVAD. Excludes requirement for IABP.
PGD-RV	Diagnosis requires either both i and ii, or iii alone:	i. Hemodynamics with RAP >15 mm Hg, PCWP <15 mm Hg, CI <2.0 L/min/m² ii. TPG <15 mm Hg and/or pulmonary artery systolic pressure <50 mm Hg, or iii. Need for RVAD

Abbreviations: BiVAD, biventricular assist device; CI, cardiac index; ECMO, extracorporeal membrane oxygenation; IABP, intraaortic balloon pump; LV, left ventricle; LVAD, left ventricular assist device; MAP, mean arterial pressure; PCWP, pulmonary capillary wedge pressure; PGD, primary graft dysfunction; RAP, right atrial pressure; RV, right ventricle; RVAD, right ventricular assist device; TPG, transpulmonary pressure gradient.

[a] Inotrope score ¼ dopamine (×1) + dobutamine (×1) + amrinone (×1)+ milrinone (×15) + epinephrine (×100) + norepinephrine (×100) with each drug dosed in μg/kg/min.

Adapted from Kobashigawa J, Zuckermann A, Macdonald P, et al. Report from a consensus conference on primary graft dysfunction after cardiac transplantation. J Heart Lung Transplant 2014;33(4):337; with permission.

Preserving and Assessing Expanded Criteria Donor Hearts for Transplantation (EXPAND; NCT02323321) will offer further insight on the impact of this platform on the incidence of PGD.

Sensitization

Not only are current heart transplant recipients older and more likely to have mechanical circulatory support, but they are also more likely to be sensitized (ie, have preformed antibodies against HLAs). Risk factors for sensitization include pregnancy, transfusions, VADs, or prior transplantation. Such preformed antibodies may cause hyperacute rejection, increase the risk of rejection posttransplantation,[17] and predispose patients to the development of cardiac allograft vasculopathy.[18]

Detection of Anti-HLA Antibodies

Currently, the detection of anti-HLA antibodies is performed most commonly using solid phase assays. With these assays, latex beads bound with single HLAs are mixed with patient serum. Antibodies will bind to their respective antigen-coated beads, are tagged with an anti-immunoglobulin G fluorescent carrier, and then detected by flow cytometry. In this manner, the identity and quantification of anti-HLA antibodies is accomplished. Quantification is important, because antibodies of greater intensity in vitro are considered to be potentially more cytotoxic in vivo. The presence of anti-HLA antibodies in high levels (usually median fluorescent intensity of >3000–5000) are considered potentially cytotoxic.[18]

Box 2
RADIAL score for assessment of primary graft dysfunction

Recipient factors

Right atrial pressure greater than 10 mm Hg

Age greater than 60 years

Diabetes

Inotrope dependence

Donor factors

Age greater than 30 years

Length of ischemic time greater than 240 minutes

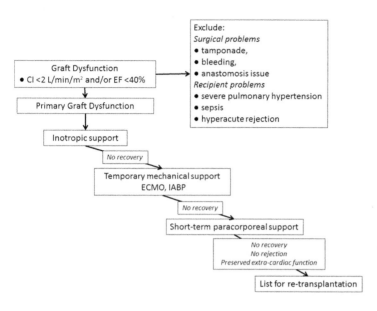

Fig. 4. Management of primary graft dysfunction (PGD). The first step in the management of PGD is to exclude treatable/reversible causes. Once surgical and recipient factors have been excluded, the treatment is supportive. For select patients with refractory graft dysfunction and preserved end-organ function, urgent listing for retransplantation may be considered, although outcomes are worse. ECMO, extracorporeal membrane oxygenation; EF, ejection fraction; IABP, intraaortic balloon pump.

However, the intensity of antibodies may not be the best test of potential cytotoxicity, because not all antibodies at high intensity may be detrimental to graft function. As newer studies indicate, the ability of donor-specific antibodies to fix complement, a functional assay may be a better marker of their cytotoxicity.[19,20] Activation of the classical complement pathway by antibodies begins with their binding of C1q, the first component of the pathway. Once activated by C1q, the classical pathway leads to the formation of the membrane attack complex and ultimately results in cell lysis and death. Thus, one would expect that antibodies with the ability to bind C1q would be more likely to be cytotoxic and this has been borne out in renal transplant recipients.[19,21] For centers where the C1q assay is not currently available, considering only antibodies that are strong binding by median fluorescent intensity (MFI) after a 1:8 or 1:16 dilution may offer comparable information.[20]

Fig. 5 outlines 1 approach to the detection of anti-HLA antibodies in heart transplant candidates and how the presence of such antibodies would change management for patients awaiting transplantation.

Approach to the Crossmatch

The detection of anti-HLA antibodies before transplantation is important, because one would avoid donors who have HLA corresponding to high-level anti-HLA antibodies in the potential recipient, as this would be a risk for hyperacute rejection. In the past, the only way to assess for this was with a

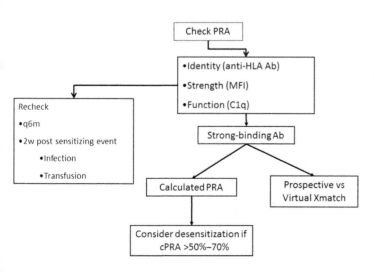

Fig. 5. Management of the sensitized patient. Sensitized patients are those with a positive panel-reactive antibody (PRA) screen. The next step is to determine the identity and intensity of the anti-HLA antibodies. This information can be used for the virtual crossmatch and to determine the calculated PRA. If the calculated PRA is above 50% to 70%, desensitization therapy may be used. cPRA, calculated panel-reactive antibody; PRA, panel-reactive antibody; MFI, median fluorescent intensity. (*From* Kittleson MM, Kobashigawa JA. Antibody-mediated rejection. Curr Opin Organ Transplant 2012;17(5):552; with permission.)

prospective crossmatch, in which the potential recipient's serum was mixed with donor cells to assess for complement-dependent cytotoxicity. However, this requirement severely geographically restricted the donor pool to hospitals near where the candidate's serum was stored, thus reducing the number of potential donors for this patient. Currently, the virtual crossmatch has replaced the prospective crossmatch at most centers. With the virtual crossmatch, HLA corresponding with high-level anti-HLA antibodies in the transplant candidate are listed as "avoids" in the United Network of Organ Sharing database, and, thus, potential donors with such HLA are not considered. This method has proven safe and successful in heart transplantation.[22] Ultimately, however, the major decision is which HLA to avoid. For those recipients with many high-level HLA antibodies, one may choose only to avoid the HLA corresponding with the very highest intensity (or complement-biding) antibodies to allow for consideration of all potential donors. Choosing to avoid HLA corresponding with only the most potentially cytotoxic anti-HLA antibodies in the virtual crossmatch would broaden the donor pool, potentially at the expense of delayed hyperacute rejection and thus this approach is often reserved only for unstable candidates unable to tolerate a long wait time to transplantation.

The Calculated Panel-Reactive Antibody

The identity and intensity of anti-HLA antibodies is useful not only in safely finding a donor organ for a sensitized recipient, but also in deciding on which sensitized patients require treatment before transplantation.[17,18] Centers often use a threshold of the calculated panel-reactive antibody (cPRA) to decide on treatment of the sensitized patient. The cPRA is the frequency of unacceptable HLA in the donor population.[23] It is computed based on HLA frequencies of 12,000 kidney donors in the United States between 2003 and 2005. For example, if a heart transplant candidate had high-level antibodies against common HLA, the cPRA might be 90%, and, thus, only 10% of all potential donors would be compatible. On the other hand, if a heart transplant candidate had only high-level antibodies against rare HLA, the cPRA might be 10%, and, thus, 90% of all potential donors would be compatible. The cPRA highlights the fact that some high-level anti-HLA antibodies will impact the ability to find a suitable donor heart more than others.[24] As with deciding on which HLA to avoid when listing a patient for transplantation, the decision about which HLA to include in the cPRA computation must balance the risks of

delayed hyperacute rejection with the risks of a prolonged wait time to transplantation. The more antibodies that are included, the higher the cPRA will be. If the cPRA is above 50% to 70%, therapies to reduce antibody levels before transplantation may be used.

Approach to Desensitization

Management of the sensitized patient involves protocols to target antibodies by inactivation (intravenous immune globulin [IV Ig][25]), removal (plasmapheresis), and decreased production (rituximab[25] and bortezomib[26]). Production of IV Ig begins with pooled human plasma from several thousand screened volunteer donors, from which highly purified polyvalent immunoglobulin G is derived. Although the mechanisms of action are incompletely understood, IV Ig suppresses inflammatory and immune-mediated processes. Side effects of IV Ig include volume overload and renal dysfunction related to the osmotic load of the sucrose additive, which may be reduced with sucrose-free preparations. Unlike other desensitization therapies, IV Ig does not increase the risk of infections.

Rituximab is a monoclonal antibody directed against the CD20 antigen on B lymphocytes. It is most commonly used for B-cell lymphoma but, in conjunction with IV Ig, also reduces HLA antibodies in patients awaiting kidney transplantation. Side effects of rituximab include a systemic inflammatory response during infusion, gastrointestinal upset, and an increase risk of infections. At our center, we use a modified protocol based on one established for desensitization of kidney transplant recipients (**Fig. 6**).[25]

If the protocol of IV Ig and rituximab is ineffective in reducing the cPRA to less than 50%, or if a patient requires rapid desensitization (ie, they are listed status 1A), then one may use bortezomib, a proteasome inhibitor against plasma cells (**Fig. 7**). It is most commonly used for the treatment of multiple myeloma, but also reduces HLA antibodies in patients awaiting heart transplantation.[26] Side effects of bortezomib include peripheral neuropathy that is usually self-limited, an increased risk of infections, and a systemic inflammatory response during infusion. To increase effectiveness, bortezomib can be combined with plasmapheresis over a 2-week cycle with plasmapheresis on the day before and day of bortezomib administration (days 0, 1, 3, 4, 7, 8, 10, and 11).

Eculizumab

Pretransplant interventions with IV Ig, rituximab, and bortezomib can reduce antibody levels such that it

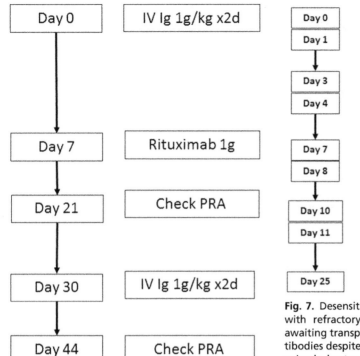

Fig. 6. Desensitization protocol. The treatment of circulating antibodies depends on the calculated panel-reactive antibody (cPRA). Treatment is considered for those patients with cPRA greater than 50% to 70%. For status 2 patients, desensitization using intravenous immunoglobulin (IV Ig) and rituximab is typically used. (Data from Vo AA, Lukovsky M, Toyoda M, et al. Rituximab and intravenous immune globulin for desensitization during renal transplantation. N Engl J Med 2008;359:242–51.)

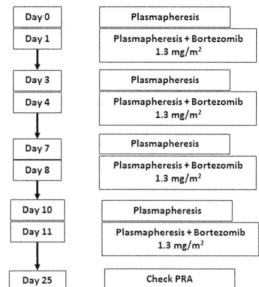

Fig. 7. Desensitization of status 1A patients or those with refractory antibodies. For status 1A patients awaiting transplantation, or those with refractory antibodies despite intravenous immunoglobulin and rituximab, bortezomib is used. This regimen will lower antibodies more effectively in these patients. PRA, panel-reactive antibody. (From Kittleson MM, Kobashigawa JA. Management of the highly sensitized patient awaiting heart transplant. Available at: http://www.acc.org/latest-in-cardiology/articles/2014/12/22/17/07/management-of-the-highly-sensitized-patient-awaiting-heart-transplant-expert-analysis. Accessed January 5, 2016.)

is possible to find an acceptable donor. However, hyperacute rejection at the time of transplantation related to preformed cytotoxic anti-HLA antibodies can still occur owing to donor-specific antibodies that were considered unlikely to be cytotoxic by virtual crossmatch or that formed after banked blood was collected for a prospective crossmatch. In this setting, eculizumab offers further insurance and protection against hyperacute rejection.

Eculizumab is a monoclonal antibody that selectively inhibits the terminal portion of the complement cascade. The complement cascade is activated by antigen–antibody complexes and ultimately leads to formation of the membrane attack complex, culminating in cell death. Eculizumab specifically binds to the terminal complement component 5, or C5, and ultimately prevents the generation of the terminal complement complex C5b-9. Eculizumab is approved by the US Food and Drug Administration for use in paroxysmal nocturnal hemoglobunuria and atypical hemolytic-uremic syndrome, 2 complement-mediated conditions. However, benefit has been seen in sensitized kidney transplant recipients.[27]

Based on the promising results in kidney transplant recipients, the De-novo Use of Eculizumab alongside Conventional Therapy in Presensitized Patients Receiving Cardiac Transplantation: An Open-Label, Investigator-Initiated Pilot (DUET; NCT02013037) study is currently ongoing at Cedars-Sinai Medical Center. In this trial, eculizumab is administered to de novo heart transplant recipients with a cPRA of greater than 70%. The primary endpoint is the incidence of antibody-mediated rejection (defined as histologic and immunopathologic evidence of antibody-related injury on endomyocardial biopsy specimens) or left ventricular dysfunction in the first 6 months after transplantation. Eculizumab increases the risk of meningococcal meningitis and patients must receive the meningococcal vaccine before administration and also receive antibiotic prophylaxis with ciprofloxacin during the 2 months of eculizumab administration.

SUMMARY

As we continue to expand the boundaries of heart transplantation to higher risk patients who are older, with mechanical circulatory support, and antibody sensitization, the goal must be to maintain superior outcomes with this scarce resource. Challenges remain in the management of heart transplant recipients, including the scarce supply and equitable distribution of donor hearts, prevention of PGD, and management of sensitization. The advances outlined in this article, from revision of the heart transplant allocation policy, a better understanding of PGD, and advances in the identification and treatment of sensitized heart transplant candidates, will serve to improve the survival and quality of life of end-stage patients who undergo heart transplantation.

REFERENCES

1. Hunt SA, Abraham WT, Chin MH, et al. 2009 focused update incorporated into the ACC/AHA 2005 guidelines for the diagnosis and management of heart failure in adults: a report of the American College of Cardiology Foundation/American Heart Association task force on practice guidelines: developed in collaboration with the international society for heart and lung transplantation. Circulation 2009;119:e391.
2. Yancy CW, Jessup M, Bozkurt B, et al. 2013 ACCF/AHA guideline for the management of heart failure: a report of the American College of Cardiology Foundation/American Heart Association Task force on practice guidelines. Circulation 2013; 128(16):e240–327.
3. Fang JC, Ewald GA, Allen LA, et al. Advanced (stage D) heart failure: a statement from the heart failure society of America guidelines committee. J Card Fail 2015;21:519.
4. Lund LH, Edwards LB, Kucheryavaya AY, et al. The registry of the international society for heart and lung transplantation: Thirty-Second Official Adult Heart Transplantation Report-2015; focus theme: early graft failure. J Heart Lung Transplant 2015;34:1244.
5. Colvin-Adams M, Smith JM, Heubner BM, et al. OPTN/SRTR 2013 annual data report: heart. Am J Transplant 2015;15(Suppl 2):1.
6. Eckman PM, Hanna M, Taylor DO, et al. Management of the sensitized adult heart transplant candidate. Clin Transplant 2010;24:726.
7. Nwakanma LU, Williams JA, Weiss ES, et al. Influence of pretransplant panel-reactive antibody on outcomes in 8,160 heart transplant recipients in recent era. Ann Thorac Surg 2007;84:1556.
8. Colvin-Adams M, Valapour M, Hertz M, et al. Lung and heart allocation in the united states. Am J Transplant 2012;12:3213.
9. Schulze PC, Kitada S, Clerkin K, et al. Regional differences in recipient waitlist time and pre- and post-transplant mortality after the 2006 united network for organ sharing policy changes in the donor heart allocation algorithm. JACC Heart Fail 2014;2:166.
10. Meyer DM, Rogers JG, Edwards LB, et al. The future direction of the adult heart allocation system in the united states. Am J Transplant 2015;15:44.
11. Kobashigawa JA, Johnson M, Rogers J, et al. Report from a forum on us heart allocation policy. Am J Transplant 2015;15:55.
12. Kobashigawa J, Patel J, Azarbal B, et al. Randomized pilot trial of gene expression profiling versus heart biopsy in the first year after heart transplant: early invasive monitoring attenuation through gene expression trial. Circ Heart Fail 2015;8:557.
13. Kobashigawa J, Zuckermann A, Macdonald P, et al. Report from a consensus conference on primary graft dysfunction after cardiac transplantation. J Heart Lung Transplant 2014;33:327.
14. Cosio Carmena MD, Gomez Bueno M, Almenar L, et al. Primary graft failure after heart transplantation: characteristics in a contemporary cohort and performance of the radial risk score. J Heart Lung Transplant 2013;32:1187.
15. Segovia J, Cosio MD, Barcelo JM, et al. Radial: a novel primary graft failure risk score in heart transplantation. J Heart Lung Transplant 2011;30:644.
16. Ardehali A, Esmailian F, Deng M, et al. Ex-vivo Perfusion of Donor Hearts for Human Heart Transplantation (PROCEED II): a prospective, open-label, multicentre, randomised non-inferiority trial. Lancet 2015;385:2577.
17. Kobashigawa J, Mehra M, West L, et al. Report from a consensus conference on the sensitized patient awaiting heart transplantation. J Heart Lung Transplant 2009;28:213.
18. Kobashigawa J, Crespo-Leiro MG, Ensminger SM, et al. Report from a consensus conference on antibody-mediated rejection in heart transplantation. J Heart Lung Transplant 2011;30:252.
19. Loupy A, Lefaucheur C, Vernerey D, et al. Complement-binding anti-HLA antibodies and kidney-allograft survival. N Engl J Med 2013;369: 1215.
20. Zeevi A, Lunz J, Feingold B, et al. Persistent strong anti-HLA antibody at high titer is complement binding and associated with increased risk of antibody-mediated rejection in heart transplant recipients. J Heart Lung Transplant 2013;32:98.
21. Sutherland SM, Chen G, Sequeira FA, et al. Complement-fixing donor-specific antibodies identified by a novel c1q assay are associated with allograft loss. Pediatr Transplant 2012;16:12.

22. Stehlik J, Islam N, Hurst D, et al. Utility of virtual crossmatch in sensitized patients awaiting heart transplantation. J Heart Lung Transplant 2009;28: 1129.

23. Cecka JM. Calculated PRA (cPRA): the new measure of sensitization for transplant candidates. Am J Transplant 2010;10:26.

24. Cecka JM, Kucheryavaya AY, Reinsmoen NL, et al. Calculated PRA: initial results show benefits for sensitized patients and a reduction in positive crossmatches. Am J Transplant 2011; 11:719.

25. Vo AA, Lukovsky M, Toyoda M, et al. Rituximab and intravenous immune globulin for desensitization during renal transplantation. N Engl J Med 2008; 359:242.

26. Patel J, Everly M, Chang D, et al. Reduction of alloantibodies via proteosome inhibition in cardiac transplantation. J Heart Lung Transplant 2011;30: 1320.

27. Stegall MD, Diwan T, Raghavaiah S, et al. Terminal complement inhibition decreases antibody-mediated rejection in sensitized renal transplant recipients. Am J Transplant 2011;11:2405.

Cardiac Resynchronization Therapy and Implantable Cardioverter Defibrillator Therapy in Advanced Heart Failure

Anthony J. Choi, MD[a], Sunu S. Thomas, MD, MSc[b],
Jagmeet P. Singh, MD, DPhil[a],*

KEYWORDS

- Heart failure • CIED • Defibrillator • Cardiac resynchronization therapy • Arrhythmia

KEY POINTS

- Cardiac implanted electronic devices (CIED) have improved survival and quality of life in patients with advanced heart failure.
- The role of implantable cardioverter defibrillators (ICD) has expanded. As clinical experience with ICDs matures, targeted antitachycardia therapies demonstrate survival and quality of life benefit.
- Cardiac resynchronization therapy addresses electrical dyssynchrony, can reverse pathologic remodeling of the left ventricle, and improves quality of life scores, measures of functional capacity, and survival.
- Although the presence of ventricular arrhythmia can portend poorer outcomes, the role and long-term management of CIEDs remains to be determined.

INTRODUCTION

Patients with heart failure represent a significant clinical and financial burden to the US health care system. In 2012, the prevalence of heart failure in the United States was 2.4%.[1] Among patients older than 80 years of age, the prevalence of heart failure is 12%. The lifetime risk of developing heart failure is 1 in 9 males and 1 in 6 for females.[2] Projections estimate that by 2030 more than 8 million people will have heart failure and the annual direct costs for heart failure care will increase to $53 billion dollars.[1] Advanced heart failure, as defined in this article, refers to patients with New York Heart Association (NYHA) functional class III or IV symptoms, inclusive of patients with American College of Cardiology/American Heart Association stage D heart failure who are listed for cardiac transplant or living with mechanical circulatory support. Fortunately, survival has improved over time, but this is overshadowed by the sobering mortality rate of 50% within 5 years of heart failure diagnosis.[3]

[a] Electrophysiology Laboratory, Cardiac Arrhythmia Service, Cardiology Division, Department of Medicine, Massachusetts General Hospital, Harvard Medical School, 55 Fruit Street, Boston, MA 02114, USA; [b] Heart Failure & Transplant Services, Cardiology Division, Department of Medicine, Massachusetts General Hospital, Harvard Medical School, 55 Fruit Street, Boston, MA 02114, USA
* Corresponding author.
E-mail address: JSINGH@mgh.harvard.edu

Heart Failure Clin 12 (2016) 423–436
http://dx.doi.org/10.1016/j.hfc.2016.03.010
1551-7136/16/$ – see front matter © 2016 Elsevier Inc. All rights reserved.

Cardiac implantable electronic devices include the implantable cardioverter-defibrillator (ICD) and cardiac resynchronization therapy (CRT) devices. These devices play an increasing role in heart failure management and have been shown to significantly improve long-term clinical outcomes in patients with moderate to severe heart failure symptoms (**Fig. 1**).

The role of ICD and CRT therapy has continually expanded. Data from quality improvement registries such as the Get With The Guidelines Heart Failure program has demonstrated an overall increase of ICD use among eligible patients from 30% to 50%.[4] Although the trend of appropriate ICD implantation is promising, it also suggests a large undertreated group of heart failure patients to whom greater effort must be directed so as to narrow the therapeutic gap among those patients for whom such devices are indicated. Patients with advanced heart failure can have limited 1-year survival and are

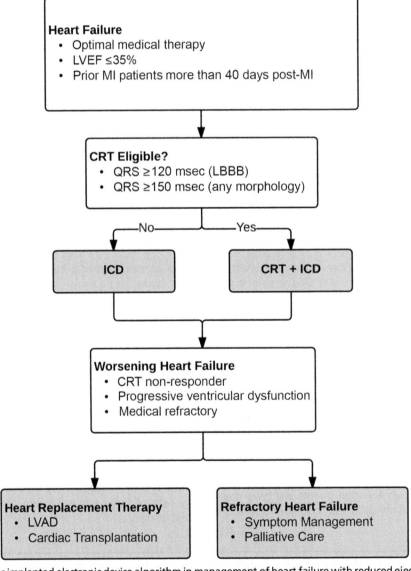

Fig. 1. Cardiac implanted electronic device algorithm in management of heart failure with reduced ejection fraction. Initial evaluation starts with identification of patients who benefit from implantable cardioverter defibrillator (ICD) for primary prevention. These patients should be on optimal medical therapy as part of their treatment strategy. A waiting period of 40 days applies for patients who have a reduced ejection fraction as a result of a myocardial infarction before they qualify for an ICD. Patients with wide QRS duration should be considered for a cardiac resynchronization therapy (CRT). LBBB, left bundle branch block; LVAD, left ventricular assist device; LVEF, left ventricular ejection fraction; MI, myocardial infarction.

frequently frail or have comorbidities that may limit their functional capacity. Guidelines recommend against implantation of ICD and CRT devices in patients where meaningful 1-year survival is not expected.[5]

IMPLANTABLE CARDIOVERTER-DEFIBRILLATORS
Background Data and Indications

ICD use was initially established as a secondary prevention strategy against sudden cardiac death. The first, largest, and frequently cited study for secondary prevention was the Antiarrhythmic versus Implantable Defibrillators (AVID) trial that found a significant survival benefit (75.4% vs 64.1% at 3 years after randomization) in patients with ICDs versus patients treated with antiarrhythmic medications (97% amiodarone or 3% with sotalol). This multicenter study enrolled 1016 patients who had either survived cardiac arrest or had sustained ventricular tachycardia with symptoms or hemodynamic compromise. In this study, the ejection fraction (EF) was an average of 32% in the ICD arm and about one-half had clinical heart failure. Despite the low average EF in this study, only 7% in the ICD group had NYHA functional class III heart failure and no patients were identified as having NYHA functional class IV heart failure.[6] A metaanalysis from the pooled data from AVID, the Cardiac Arrest Study Hamburg,[7] and the Canadian Implantable Defibrillator Study[8] found that ICD therapy resulted in a significant relative reduction in overall mortality (28%) and mortality identified owing to arrhythmia (50%). In this pooled database, the average EF was less than 35% in both the ICD and antiarrhythmic treatment groups. Despite this low EF, patients with NYHA functional class II or greater symptoms were not well-represented in either the ICD or amiodarone treatment arms (9% and 12%, respectively).[9]

Because survival in patients with cardiac arrest is poor,[10–13] there has been interest in identifying patients who would benefit from implantation of an ICD on a primary prevention basis.

The Multicenter Automatic Defibrillator Implantation Trial (MADIT) compared ICDs with conventional therapy in patients with EF of 35% or greater, nonsustained ventricular tachycardia, and NYHA functional class I to III heart failure. Eligible patients were referred for an electrophysiologic study and were randomized to antiarrhythmic treatment; the majority was treated with amiodarone (73%). The study was terminated after enrollment of 196 patients after preliminary analysis demonstrated a reduced rate of all-cause mortality of 38.6% in the antiarrhythmic therapy

group and 15.8% in the defibrillator group with a hazard ratio (HR) of 0.46 (P = .009).[14]

MADIT II directly addressed concerns from the first MADIT study, namely an absence of a conventional therapy arm, higher percentage of patients on beta-blockers in the ICD group, and lifted the requirement for an electrophysiologic study to guide enrollment. In this study, patients with prior myocardial infarction and an EF of less than 30% were randomized to a control group and an ICD group. The use of class I antiarrhythmic drugs was minimal in this study when compared with MADIT (13% in both arms in MADIT vs <1% in either group in MADIT II) and the use of beta-blockers was 70% in both arms. Mortality in the ICD arm was found to be 14.2% compared with 19.8% in the control group (HR, 0.69; P = .016). Another landmark study, Sudden Cardiac Death in Heart Failure Trial, randomized 2521 patients with NYHA functional class II and III heart failure and a left ventricular (LV) EF (LVEF) of 35% or less with conventional therapy versus amiodarone versus ICD therapy. This was the first study to also include patients with nonischemic cardiomyopathy. Overall, ICD therapy was superior in terms of the primary endpoint (5-year event rate, 28.9%) versus amiodarone and placebo arms (34.0% and 36.1%, respectively). Nonischemic and ischemic heart failure had similar benefit of ICD therapy on mortality (HR, 0.73 and 0.79; P = .06 and P = .05; both respectively). This study also demonstrated that amiodarone was not better than placebo with regard to mortality.[15]

For patients with NYHA functional class IV, stage D heart failure, it is important to consider that heart failure treatment trials have shown that with worsening NYHA functional class, there is a shift in the cause of death from arrhythmia to pump failure. The Effect of metoprolol CR/XL in chronic heart failure: Metoprolol CR/XL Randomised Intervention Trial in Congestive Heart Failure (MERIT-HF) trial found that the most common mode of death was attributed to sudden death in patients with NYHA functional class II and III heart failure (84% and 59%, respectively), which then shifted to progressive pump failure (56%) in patients with NYHA IV symptoms, with a minority still suffering from sudden cardiac death (33%).[16]

Tachyarrhythmia Detection and Therapy

Understanding the basic programming features for ICDs is important for the heart failure physician. As implantation of primary prevention ICDs has increased, so have concerns for increased defibrillator therapies for both appropriate and inappropriate events. Patients who experience defibrillator therapy can exhibit anxiety, depression, and measurable changes in quality of life measures.[17,18] Data from the MADIT II study has also demonstrated that inappropriate shocks were associated with an increased likelihood of all-cause mortality (HR, 2.29; $P = .025$).[19] Antitachycardia pacing as a therapeutic modality has not been shown convincingly to have a similar detrimental effect on survival.[20]

One approach to reducing the number of defibrillator therapies is to increase the duration of the detection criteria with the hypothesis that this would reduce inappropriate shocks and allow for ventricular tachycardia to self-terminate. This was first reported in the Prevention Parameters Evaluation (PREPARE) study, which looked at patients who were implanted with a CRT-D or ICD for primary prevention within the preceding 6 months of enrollment and without episodes of ventricular tachycardia. A total of 700 patients were programmed to prolonged detection duration (30 out of 40 beats) and the outcomes were compared with a combined control group composed of historical controls from the Multicenter InSync Randomized Clinical Evaluation (MIRACLE)[21] trial and the Comparison of Empiric to Physician-Tailored Programming of Implantable Cardioverter-Defibrillators (EMPIRIC)[22] trials. In the study arm with prolonged duration detection, 41% of patients had NYHA functional class III/IV symptoms and at the end of the 12-month follow-up, there were significantly less shocks from any cause (16.9% vs 8.5%). Additionally, there was also a reduction in the 12-month secondary endpoint of overall morbidity in the PREPARE versus the historical control group (4.9% vs 8.7%; $P<.01$). Whereas the combined control group and the PREPARE group had matched age, gender, and NYHA functional class, there were statistically significant differences in the baseline characteristics between the 2 groups. Despite fewer shocks being delivered to the patient the group with extended ventricular tachycardia detection criteria, they did not experience adverse outcomes.[23]

MIRACLE and EMPIRIC were followed by a controlled study: Role Of Long Detection Window Programming In Patients With Left Ventricular Dysfunction, Non-Ischemic Etiology In Primary Prevention Treated With A Biventricular ICD (RELEVANT). A total of 883 patients were enrolled and 1 group was programmed with extended detection criteria similar to the PREPARE programming of 30 out of 40 beats as opposed to the 12 of 16 beats in the control arm. This study had an average NYHA functional class of 2.67 in both groups and all other characteristics were well-matched. Patients were

followed for an average of 36 months. Those patients in the extended detection arm were found to have benefit with improved freedom from appropriate and inappropriate first shocks and favorable reductions in heart failure hospitalizations in the study group.[24]

The Reduction in Inappropriate Therapy and Mortality through ICD Programming (MADIT-RIT) study reflected further endeavors to determine optimal programming that would both reduce obligatory shocks after either inappropriate antitachycardia pacing or inappropriate shocks without adverse consequence to morbidity or mortality. A total of 1500 patients were enrolled who included patients who had either ischemic or nonischemic heart failure and met approved primary prevention guidelines for ICD or CRT-D. The study randomized these patients to a conventional therapy arm, a high rate arm, and a duration-delay arm. Endpoints of this study were defined as first occurrence of inappropriate therapy, death, or first episode of syncope. After a mean follow-up period of 1.4 years, the duration-delay group was noted to have a reduction in the first shock for inappropriate therapy by 76% when compared with the conventional therapy arm (HR, 0.24; $P<.001$). Also observed was a reduction in the frequency of initial inappropriate shocks in the high-rate therapy arm (HR, 0.21; $P<.001$). No difference in mortality and first episode of syncope was found in either conventional treatment or either study arms.[25] Importantly, this study showed that long-term outcomes were significantly better in the arms with delayed programming or a high rate cutoff.

Thus, for primary prevention patients, the recent 2015 HRS/EHRA/APHRS/SOLAECE Expert Consensus Statement on Optimal Implantable Cardioverter-Defibrillator Programming and Testing guidelines recommend tachyarrhythmia detection duration criteria require 6 to 12 seconds or 30 intervals before completing detection (class IA) and that the slowest therapy zone be limited to tachycardias between 185 and 200 bpm (class IA) as to reduce total therapies.[26]

In summary, the role of ICD therapy in advanced heart failure continues to expand. It is important to pay attention to programming these devices, because it can have a significant impact on short- and long-term clinical outcomes.

CARDIAC RESYNCHRONIZATION THERAPY

In contrast with the ICD, where survival benefit is driven by prevention of sudden death in the heart failure population, biventricular pacing results in an improvement of quality of life, functional scores, and survival.[21,27]

Electrical activation sequence determines the coordinated cardiac contraction and relaxation cycle. Patients with abnormal activation sequences, notably those with an intraventricular conduction defect, exhibit electrical dyssynchrony. In the setting of a left bundle branch block (LBBB) pattern, mechanical dyssynchrony manifests as the activation wave front results in the early activation of the septum causing an early mechanical shortening of the septum followed by delayed activation of the lateral LV wall. Strain analysis demonstrates LV mechanical stretch during early systole with subsequent contraction of the prestretched myocardium during the delayed LV activation (**Fig. 2**). Locally, this area of the LV wall may be characterized by pathologic changes in mitochondrial functioning,[28,29] calcium handling,[30] and β-adrenergic reserve.[31] The delayed activation of the lateral LV wall may result in increased oxygen consumption and reduced LV contractile efficiency. Furthermore, improvements in mechanical contraction may mirror improvements in electrical synchrony that are seen from LV or biventricular pacing.[32]

Landmark Trials in Cardiac Resynchronization Therapy

Early studies of CRT in heart failure patients were limited to patients in NYHA functional class III or

higher. The first of the large-scale trials was the Multisite Stimulation in Cardiomyopathy (MUSTIC) trial. This was a cross-over study in which 67 patients with NYHA functional class III heart failure, QRS interval of 150 ms or greater, an LVEF of less than 0.35, and an LV end diastolic diameter of greater than 60 mm were randomized in a blinded fashion to an active arm with biventricular pacing turned on and a control arm with biventricular pacing turned off. After 12 weeks, the groups were switched and in both arms (inactive to active vs active to inactive) CRT was notable for improvements in 6M walk distance (6MWD), peak oxygen consumption (pVO$_2$) and quality of life scores, and significant decrease in heart failure hospitalizations.[33]

Following the European studies of CRT, the first in the United States was the Multicenter InSync Randomized Clinical Evaluation (MIRACLE). This was a prospective, randomized, double-blind trial in patients with NYHA functional class III or IV, a LVEF of 0.35 or less, an LV end diastolic diameter of 55 mm or greater, and a QRS interval of 130 ms or greater. In this study, patients with a pacing indication were not included and required optimal medical therapy (OMT). Four hundred fifty-three patients were randomized to OMT without CRT versus OMT with CRT. CRT resulted in improvements in NYHA functional class, 6MWD, and quality of life, and decreased hospitalizations.

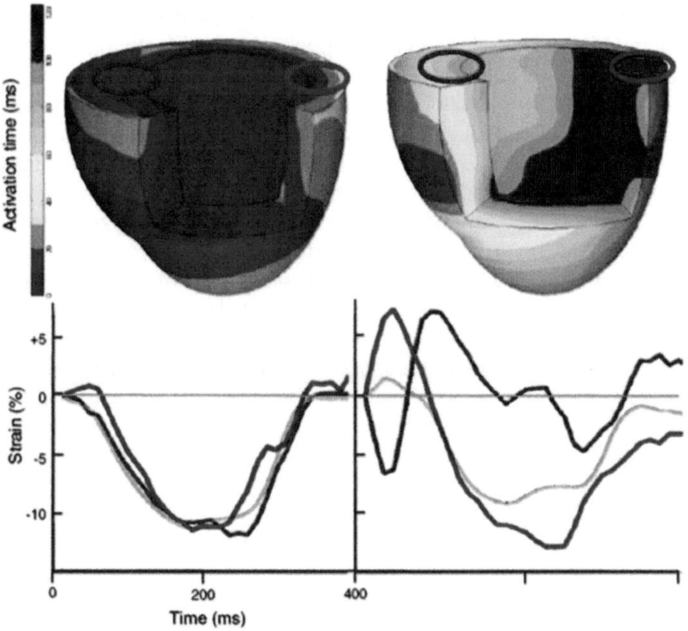

Fig. 2. Relationship between electrical and mechanical dyssynchrony in left bundle branch block (LBBB). The top panels are a colorimetric representation of myocardial activation. The blue circles mark the septal activation and the red circles mark the lateral left ventricular (LV) wall. The bottom panels show strain of the septum (*blue line*) and lateral LV wall (*red line*). The left panels represent normal activation and the right panels represent LBBB activation. Activation time in LBBB is earliest in the septum with significant delay of the lateral LV wall (*top right panel*) in contrast with nearly simultaneous activation of the LV (*top left panel*). Strain analysis of the myocardium in LBBB demonstrates early shortening of the septum with mechanical stretch of the lateral LV wall in early systole with subsequent shortening in late systole (*bottom right panel*). This is in contrast with coordinated septal and lateral LV wall shortening in normal electrical activation (*bottom left panel*). (*From* Prinzen FW, Vernooy K, De Boeck BW, et al. Mechano-energetics of the asynchronous and resynchronized heart. Heart Fail Rev 2011;16(3):215–24.)

Reversal of ventricular remodeling was demonstrated by improved LVEF, and reduction in LV end diastolic diameter and severity of mitral regurgitation.[21]

A similar comparison was performed in Europe in the Cardiac Resynchronization on Morbidity and Mortality in Heart Failure (CARE-HF) trial with similar inclusion criteria to the MIRACLE study, but unlike previous studies, CARE-HF included patients with a QRS interval of greater than 120 ms so long as patients with borderline electrical dyssynchrony of 120 to 150 ms demonstrated dyssynchrony by echocardiography. Similar findings of improvement of cardiac function, quality of life, and reduction of hospitalizations were observed. Follow-up at 18 months showed that patients in the CRT group (n = 409) improved from NYHA functional class III/IV symptoms to NYHA functional class I (in 37%) and class II (37%).[34] Follow-up to 30 months demonstrated a 40% reduction of death and heart failure hospitalization and 36% reduction in all-cause mortality.[35]

Efficacy trials for the effectiveness of CRT were coincident with studies demonstrating efficacy of ICD for primary prevention of sudden death in patients with heart failure and reduced EF. The Comparison of Medical Therapy, Pacing and Defibrillation in Heart Failure (COMPANION) study randomized 1520 patients with NYHA functional class III or IV symptoms, LVEF of 0.35 or less, QRS interval of 120 ms or greater, and PR of greater than 150 ms without indication for pacing to a 3-arm study in a 1:2:2 fashion (OMT, OMT + CRT-P, OMT + CRT-D). Compared with OMT alone, both CRT-P and CRT-D significantly reduced the risk of death or heart failure hospitalization by approximately 20%. Similarly, both CRT-P and CRT-D reduced the hazard of all-cause mortality (by 24% and 36%, respectively), although the reduction in mortality was only of borderline significance for CRT-P.[36]

Improving Response to Resynchronization Therapy

Of concern in these studies was the rate of nonresponders to CRT, which approached one-third of patients receiving the device. As the advanced heart failure population experiences a high rate of morbidity and mortality, identifying responders before implant and maximizing response to CRT is of paramount importance.

Patient selection for CRT is limited to moderate-severely reduced EF (≤35%) and QRS duration as seen on a surface electrocardiogram. Thus, the QRS duration is used as a surrogate for electrical and mechanical synchrony. In patients with a LBBB, LV activation is delayed in the basal posterior/posterolateral segment of the LV.[37] This would argue intuitively for targeting this segment for LV pacing. Patients with an intraventricular conduction defect and right bundle branch block (RBBB) have different activation patterns and may not benefit from CRT.[38] However, there is heterogeneity on activation wave fronts that are often different depending on the etiology of the cardiomyopathy (ischemic vs nonischemic). Because this creates a variable landscape a proportion of patients with RBBB and intraventricular conduction defect do indeed have significant LV delay, which may benefit potentially from biventricular pacing.[38,39] Identification of patients with RBBB or intraventricular conduction defect who may benefit from CRT is being evaluated in a prospective study with individualized targeting of the LV lead in patients with a non-LBBB morphology (ENHANCE CRT; ClinicalTrials.gov NCT01983293).

Recent North American guidelines have cited the findings of COMPANION, CARE-HF, and MADIT-CRT as rationale to restrict the class I indication for CRT therapy to patients with an LBBB. This is in agreement with findings from a metaanalysis that included the COMPANION, CARE-HF, MADIT-CRT, and RAFT studies where patients with an LBBB morphology benefited from a 40% reduction in composite events (death, heart failure admissions).[40]

Pulmonary hypertension and right ventricular (RV) failure may also predict nonresponse to CRT. Right heart catheterization and echocardiographic data from 101 CRT patients with pulmonary hypertension were analyzed in a retrospective study with primary endpoint of death and a composite endpoint of death, need for LVAD, and transplant. Patients whose transpulmonary gradient (defined as mean pulmonary artery pressure – pulmonary capillary wedge pressure) was greater than or equal to 12 mm Hg had worse primary (HR, 3.2; $P = .009$) and composite outcomes (HR, 3.0; $P = .004$). Similarly, RV dilatation (RV end diastolic dimension >42 mm) was an independent predictor for CRT nonresponse in the composite (HR, 4.2; $P = .002$) and primary endpoints (HR, 3.2; $P = .02$).[41]

Intraprocedural Optimization Strategies

The traditional target for the LV lead is based on the anatomic correlate that the posterolateral wall is frequently delayed in activation, especially in patients with LBBB. Although pacing at an anatomically favorable position can cause an immediate improvement in hemodynamics, there is variability in CRT response when the sites are chosen purely on the basis of anatomic targeting.[42] The intuitive target of CRT is to activate sites of latest electrical delay, which can be assessed using intracardiac electrograms to determine the interval between the surface QRS and earliest intracardiac signal of the LV lead.[43] This approach was evaluated retrospectively in 280 patients who met standard criteria for a CRT-D and were part of the SMART-AV study.[44] In this subgroup, the mean EF was 28% with a mean LV end systolic volume of 129 mL. Echocardiographic assessment was performed by estimating the volume in end systole and end diastole. There was a significant correlation between reduction of both volume in end systole and end diastole when compared with the onset of ventricular activation to the first peak from the LV electrogram at the site of implantation.[43]

Although anatomic and electrical timing correlate with potentially improve CRT response, patients with cardiomyopathy may have significant scar, which may not allow for pacing of the LV at the most ideal location. Given the limitations of the conventional transvenous route (**Fig. 3**), several novel pacing approaches have been considered in the patient with advanced heart failure. Alternative approaches via the endocardial and epicardial approach have the potential to enhance response in a subset of this cohort.[42,45]

Endocardial pacing may result in more physiologic depolarization of the ventricles from the endocardial surface to the epicardial surface. Endocardial pacing has shown promising results with improved clinical and LV hemodynamic parameters. The Alternate Site Cardiac Resynchronization (ALSYNC) study was performed to assess the safety and efficacy of LV endocardial pacing in 138 patients. These patients were previously deemed to have a CS approach that was technically difficult or were CRT non responders. In almost two-thirds of the study arms, clinical and echocardiographic improvement was noted.[46] In up to 10% of patients undergoing biventricular pacemaker implantation, LV lead placement is challenging for a variety of reasons, namely, an inability to cannulate the coronary sinus, absence of suitable branches, lack of lead stability, phrenic nerve capture, and so on. In such situations, surgical LV epicardial lead placement is an option with approaches to epicardial LV lead placement to include left anterior or lateral minithoracotomy, videoassisted thoracotomy, and robotic surgical systems.[47]

Postimplant Care for the Patient Undergoing Cardiac Resynchronization Therapy

Contemporary post device implant care continues to remain deficient on many fronts, namely, optimization of the AV and VV intervals, consideration of device diagnostic information along with the utilization of such data to risk stratify patients for early identification, and treatment of nonresponders. There is evidence to suggest that adjusting and

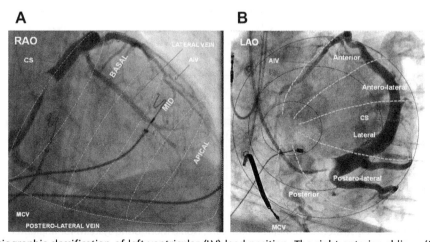

Fig. 3. Angiographic classification of left ventricular (LV) lead position. The right anterior oblique (*RAO, A*) enables segmental visualization of the long axis into the basal, mid, and apical segments of the LV. The left anterior oblique (*LAO, B*) visualizes the LV in the short axis and segments the LV into the anterior, anterolateral, lateral, posterolateral, and posterior segments. (*Adapted from* Singh JP, Klein HU, Huang DT, et al. Left ventricular lead position and clinical outcome in the Multicenter Automatic Defibrillator Implantation Trial-Cardiac Resynchronization Therapy (MADIT-CRT) trial. Circulation 2011;123(11):1159–66; with permission.)

optimizing the AV interval can result in hemodynamic benefits; however, there remains a paucity of information on the impact of this optimization on the electrical activation sequence. A substantial percentage of nonresponders to biventricular pacing may actually benefit from AV interval optimization. Whether AV optimization is necessary for each patient at the time of their device implantation is controversial. However, it seems intuitive that patients would need these intervals optimized owing to the large extent of variability in the position of the atrial, RV and LV leads. Also adding to variability are the interpatient differences in substrate and scar distribution. At this time, the data are evolving, but evidence from the SMART-AV and ADAPTIVE CRT study suggests that patients with any atrioventricular block, especially RBBB would benefit from device optimization.[48,49]

CRT devices have the ability to provide information on patient activity, heart rate, autonomic activity, and transthoracic impedance as a surrogate for pulmonary edema.[50] The use of remote monitoring has also enabled the wireless automatic transmission of ambulatory. In the setting of a well-integrated multidisciplinary team can enhance the treatment and monitoring of patients with heart failure.[51,52] With remote monitoring, parameters from biometric data can be established to detect problems early that allow for proactive adjustment of drug regimen or device settings

(Fig. 4). Although this is a promising approach, prospective studies demonstrating favorable clinical outcomes do not yet exist.

CARDIAC IMPLANTED ELECTRONIC DEVICE THERAPY IN PATIENTS WITH A LEFT VENTRICULAR ASSIST DEVICE

Patients with advanced heart failure whose symptoms are refractory to conventional drug and electrical device therapy may benefit from the use of LV assist device (LVAD) therapy. In the landmark Randomized Evaluation Of Mechanical Assistance For The Treatment Of Congestive Heart Failure (REMATCH), the most marginal of heart failure patients, ineligible for cardiac transplantation were treated with either a first generation pulsatile LVAD or OMT. The results profoundly demonstrated a significant survival benefit at 12 (52% vs 25%) and 24 months (23% vs 8%) among those treated with mechanical circulatory support.[53] In the decade following the publication of REMATCH, the field of mechanical circulatory support has witnessed the evolution of device technology with continuous axial flow (Thoratec HeartMate II)[54] and centrifugual (HeartWare HVAD) pumps,[55] and expansion of device indication to both destination therapy among transplant ineligible patients, and as a bridge to transplant[56] in those patients listed for cardiac

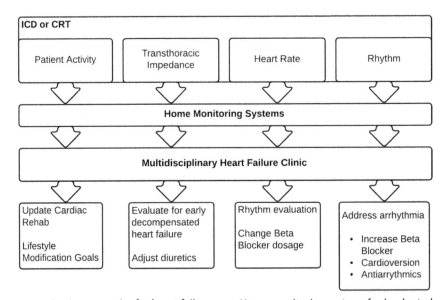

Fig. 4. Remote monitoring strategies for heart failure care. Home monitoring systems for implanted cardiac electrical devices provide remote transmission of rhythm analysis, baseline electrocardiograph, transthoracic impedance, and patient activity. Commercially available devices at home can provide patient data to upload to the Internet or can be web-connected directly. The flow of information can feed into a multidisciplinary heart failure clinic and can provide the opportunity to make adjustments to home medications (ie, beta-blockers or diuretics) or prompt a request for the patient to seek unscheduled medical evaluation. CRT, cardiac resynchronization therapy; ICD, implantable cardioverter-defibrillator.

transplant but with hemodynamics too marginal for survival to transplantation.

The current generation of LVADs has demonstrated improved survival and significant improvement of quality of life and functional measures.[54,57,58] In fact, current registry data indicate that 1-year LVAD survival[59] approximates that of cardiac transplantation[60] (80% vs 85%). The destination therapy group is the fastest growing group of LVAD patients accounting for 43% of implanted LVADs between 2011 and 2013.[61] It is expected that the number of patients with LVADs will increase with further advances in patient selection, the introduction of a new generation of devices, and the reduction in adverse events that can challenge overall survival outcomes.

Ventricular Arrhythmias in the Patient with a Left Ventricular Assist Device

Ventricular arrhythmias are most frequently detected within the first 30 days after implantation of an LVAD. In a multicenter study of 281 patients receiving a continuous flow LVAD, 13% of patients had ventricular arrhythmias within the first 30 days. After 30 days from LVAD implant, only 8% were noted to have ventricular arrhythmias.[57] A more recent single-center study of 169 patients found that 23.5% had ventricular arrhythmias in the early period with the greatest risk on postoperative day 1. Patients who had a nonischemic cardiomyopathy and had pre-LVAD ventricular arrhythmia had a greater than 2-fold risk of developing early ventricular arrhythmias. Of the patients enrolled, 129 had an active ICD, with a total of 25 shocks delivered and of those, 8 (32%) developed acute RV failure. Of the 13 patients who received antitachycardia pacing, there was no acute RV failure.[62]

The clinical implication of ventricular arrhythmias seems to be minimized by the presence of an LVAD. Of note, many patients to a significant degree can tolerate transient ventricular arrhythmias, although more prolonged ventricular arrhythmias can result in right heart failure, hemodynamic instability, ICD therapies, and mortality. Indeed, patients with early ventricular arrhythmias within 1 week of LVAD implant demonstrated an associated 5-fold higher mortality rate.[63]

The role of the ICD in patients with LVADs remains controversial. For LVAD patients in the REMATCH study, there were no deaths that were attributed to ventricular arrhythmias. Adverse events reported in this study demonstrated a nonsignificant difference in the rate per patient-years of 0.56 in the medical therapy arm to 0.25 in the LVAD group (rate ratio of 0.45

with a 95% CI of 0.22–0.90).[53] Another single-center study reviewed registry data from 478 consecutive patients who received VAD placement between 1991 and 2008. Ninety of these patients (18.8%) had an ICD at the time of implant and this cohort had a significant reduction in mortality (HR, 0.55; 95% CI. 0.32–0.94; P = .028).[64] The older period of observation explains the heterogeneous group of mechanical support modalities used (primarily pulsatile LVADs, with 7.5% right ventricular assist devices, and 5.9% biventricular assist devices). More recent experience at a different single center with a continuous flow LVADs and late ventricular arrhythmias (>30 days) observed that the postoperative risk was found to be related to the presence of preoperative arrhythmia and patients with an ICD

Box 1
ICDs with known interference with the HeartMate II left ventricular assist device[a]

- St. Jude Medical
  - Atlas-HF V-340
  - Atlas-HF V-341
  - Atlas-HF V-343
  - Atlas V193
  - Atlas V-242
  - Atlas V-243
  - Atlas V-366
  - Atlas VR model V-199
  - Current DR RF 2207-36
  - Current RF VR 1207-36
  - Epic HF CRT-D model V-337
  - Epic HF CRT-D model V-338
  - Epic HF V-350
  - Epic Plus VR model V-196
  - Integrity SR 5142
  - Photon Micron DR model V-232
  - Promote RF CRT-D model 3207-36
  - SN V-235
- Sorin
  - Alto 2 model 624

[a] List of devices for which interrogation was confounded by electromagnetic interference from the left ventricular assist device.
Data from Thoratec. Reported ICD Experience. Available at: http://www.thoratec.com/medical-professionals/reported-icd-experience.aspx. Accessed March 9, 2016.

demonstrated a subtle trend toward better cumulative survival, although this was not statistically significant with 250 days of follow-up (90.6% vs 85.6%; $P = .55$).[65]

Currently, the only guidelines that discuss the role of ICDs in LVAD patients are limited to resuming tachytherapies after implant (class I, level of evidence A), consideration of implanting an ICD for patients with LVADS who may not have an already existing ICD (class IIa, level of evidence B), and a recommendation to turn off the defibrillator in patients with biventricular VAD support and recurrent ventricular arrhythmia (class II, level of evidence C).[66] Overall, there is a relative paucity of data to direct an evidence-based approach to the implantation, maintenance, or simply allow the generator to achieve end of life without replacement.

Retrospective studies have identified the following, which should factor into the decision analysis when ICD implantation is to be considered in a prospective LVAD patient. (1) Ventricular arrhythmias are typically well-tolerated in LVAD patients, but may lead to an eventual worsening of heart failure and increase the risk for cardiac arrest. (2) Patients who receive ICD shocks tend to develop acute heart failure as opposed to patients who terminated their arrhythmia by antitachycardia pacing. (3) Patients with preexisting ventricular arrhythmias are at high risk for late ventricular arrhythmia after LVAD implantation. (4) For those patients implanted with an LVAD with a de novo or preexisting ICD or CRT device, care must be taken to ensure appropriate sensing function and avoidance of electromagnetic interference from the LVAD that could affect the functionality of the ICD. There have been case reports of inappropriate therapies owing to electromagnetic interference from a VAD.[67] Near-field telemetry is known to be affected in HeartMate II LVAD patients with St. Jude Medical and Sorin defibrillator devices (**Box 1**).[68]

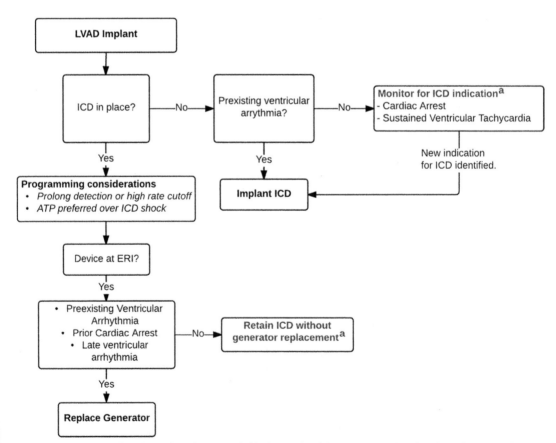

Fig. 5. Management of implanted cardioverter defibrillators (ICD) for patients treated with a left ventricular assist device (LVAD). The paradigm for cardiac arrest prevention shifts because patients with LVADs can tolerate ventricular arrhythmia. Tachycardia detection and therapy should be programmed to minimize shocks by prolonging detection times or increasing the rate cutoff for tachycardia detection. The role of maintaining an ICD in an elective replacement period (ERI) or implanting an ICD for primary prevention is controversial. ATP, Antitachycardia pacing. [a] No guideline-based recommendations exist and depends on institutional protocols.

A reasonable approach would be to retain ICDs in potential LVAD patients with preexisting ICDs. For secondary prevention, new ICD implants should be considered in patients who have demonstrated either preoperative ventricular arrhythmias or a high burden of postoperative ventricular arrhythmia. Therapy programming should make an attempt to minimize high voltage defibrillation by prolonging detect times, optimizing the use of antitachycardia pacing, and ensuring that the patient is medically optimized (**Fig. 5**). However, because data are derived mostly from LVAD implant registries, evidence-based guidance is limited.

Role of Cardiac Resynchronization Therapy in the Patient with a Left Ventricular Assist Device

The role of biventricular or LV pacing in patients with LVADs requires further elucidation. To this end, it remains to be determined as to whether resynchronization of ventricular function is of hemodynamic importance in the setting of mechanical circulatory support. A recent report in a small cohort of 61 patients with ICD or CRT-D before the LVAD implant, showed no significant survival benefit in either of the groups during follow-up. Interestingly all deaths were nonarrhythmic in the study, and there was no difference in survival between the ICD or CRT arm of the study.[69]

SUMMARY

Advanced heart failure patients benefit from implantable device therapy, either through the reduction of sudden cardiac death or an improvement of cardiac function via resynchronization therapy. Many of these patients over time continue to have progressive heart failure and become candidates for mechanical circulatory support. In recent years, a high proportion of patients with mechanical support frequently have a preexisting CRT or ICD device. There are few data on the additional benefit of continued ICD or CRT therapy in this group of patients advanced heart failure. Much work still needs to be done on exploring the benefits of individualized programming and understanding the interactions of these devices in this expanding cohort of patients.

REFERENCES

1. Heidenreich PA, Albert NM, Allen LA, et al. Forecasting the impact of heart failure in the United States: a policy statement from the American Heart Association. Circ Heart Fail 2013;6(3):606–19.

2. Lloyd-Jones DM. Lifetime risk for developing congestive heart failure: the Framingham Heart Study. Circulation 2002;106(24):3068–72.

3. Mozaffarian D, Benjamin EJ, Go AS, et al. Heart disease and stroke statistics-2015 update: a report from the American Heart Association. Circulation 2015;131(4):e29–322.

4. Hess PL, Grau-Sepulveda MV, Hernandez AF, et al. Age differences in the use of implantable cardioverter-defibrillators among older patients hospitalized with heart failure. J Cardiovasc Electrophysiol 2013;24(6):664–71.

5. Writing Committee Members, Yancy CW, Jessup M, et al. 2013 ACCF/AHA guideline for the management of heart failure: a report of the American College of Cardiology Foundation/American Heart Association Task Force on practice guidelines. Circulation 2013;128:e240–327. Lippincott Williams & Wilkins.

6. A Comparison of antiarrhythmic-drug therapy with implantable defibrillators in patients resuscitated from near-fatal ventricular arrhythmias. N Engl J Med 1997;337(22):1576–83.

7. Kuck KH, Cappato R, Siebels J, et al. Randomized comparison of antiarrhythmic drug therapy with implantable defibrillators in patients resuscitated from cardiac arrest : the Cardiac Arrest Study Hamburg (CASH). Circulation 2000;102(7):748–54.

8. Connolly SJ, Gent M, Roberts RS, et al. Canadian Implantable Defibrillator Study (CIDS) : a randomized trial of the implantable cardioverter defibrillator against amiodarone. Circulation 2000;101(11):1297–302.

9. Connolly SJ, Hallstrom AP, Cappato R, et al. Meta-analysis of the implantable cardioverter defibrillator secondary prevention trials. AVID, CASH and CIDS studies. Antiarrhythmics vs Implantable Defibrillator study. Cardiac Arrest Study Hamburg. Canadian Implantable Defibrillator Study. Eur Heart J 2000;21(24):2071–8.

10. Rea TD, Crouthamel M, Eisenberg MS, et al. Temporal patterns in long-term survival after resuscitation from out-of-hospital cardiac arrest. Circulation 2003;108(10):1196–201.

11. Wong M, Morrison LJ, Qiu F, et al. Trends in short- and long-term survival among out-of-hospital cardiac arrest patients alive at hospital arrival. Circulation 2014;130(21):1883–90.

12. de Vreede-Swagemakers J. Out-of-hospital cardiac arrest in the 1990s: a population-based study in the Maastricht area on incidence, characteristics and survival. J Am Coll Cardiol 1997;30(6):1500–5.

13. Chan PS, McNally B, Tang F, et al. Recent trends in survival from out-of-hospital cardiac arrest in the United States. Circulation 2014;130(21):1876–82.

14. Moss AJ, Hall WJ, Cannom DS, et al. Improved survival with an implanted defibrillator in patients with

coronary disease at high risk for ventricular arrhythmia. Multicenter Automatic Defibrillator Implantation Trial Investigators. N Engl J Med 1996;335(26):1933–40.

15. Bardy GH, Lee KL, Mark DB, et al. Amiodarone or an implantable cardioverter-defibrillator for congestive heart failure. N Engl J Med 2005;352(3):225–37.

16. Effect of metoprolol CR/XL in chronic heart failure: Metoprolol CR/XL Randomised Intervention Trial in-Congestive Heart Failure (MERIT-HF). Lancet 1999;353(9169):2001–7.

17. Heller SS, Ormont MA, Lidagoster L, et al. Psychosocial outcome after ICD implantation: a current perspective. Pacing Clin Electrophysiol 1998;21(6):1207–15.

18. Schron EB, Exner DV, Yao Q, et al. Quality of life in the antiarrhythmics versus implantable defibrillators trial: impact of therapy and influence of adverse symptoms and defibrillator shocks. Circulation 2002;105(5):589–94.

19. Daubert JP, Zareba W, Cannom DS, et al. Inappropriate implantable cardioverter-defibrillator shocks in MADIT II. J Am Coll Cardiol 2008;51(14):1357–65.

20. Sweeney MO, Sherfesee L, DeGroot PJ, et al. Differences in effects of electrical therapy type for ventricular arrhythmias on mortality in implantable cardioverter-defibrillator patients. Heart Rhythm 2010;7(3):353–60.

21. Abraham WT, Fisher WG, Smith AL, et al. Cardiac resynchronization in chronic heart failure. N Engl J Med 2002;346(24):1845–53.

22. Wilkoff BL, Ousdigian KT, Sterns LD, et al. A comparison of empiric to physician-tailored programming of implantable cardioverter-defibrillators: results from the prospective randomized multicenter EMPIRIC trial. J Am Coll Cardiol 2006;48(2):330–9.

23. Wilkoff BL, Williamson BD, Stern RS, et al. Strategic programming of detection and therapy parameters in implantable cardioverter-defibrillators reduces shocks in primary prevention patients. J Am Coll Cardiol 2008;52(7):541–50.

24. Gasparini M, Menozzi C, Proclemer A, et al. A simplified biventricular defibrillator with fixed long detection intervals reduces implantable cardioverter defibrillator (ICD) interventions and heart failure hospitalizations in patients with non-ischaemic cardiomyopathy implanted for primary prevention: the RELEVANT [Role of long dEtection window programming in patients with LEft VentriculAr dysfunction, Non-ischemic eTiology in primary prevention treated with a biventricular ICD] study. Eur Heart J 2009;30(22):2758–67.

25. Moss AJ, Schuger C, Beck CA, et al. Reduction in inappropriate therapy and mortality through ICD Programming. N Engl J Med 2012;367(24):2275–83.

26. Wilkoff BL, Fauchier L, Stiles MK, et al. 2015 HRS/EHRA/APHRS/SOLAECE Expert Consensus Statement on Optimal Implantable Cardioverter-Defibrillator Programming and Testing: Developed in partnership with and endorsed by the European Heart Rhythm Association (EHRA), the Asia Pacific Heart Rhythm Society (APHRS), and the Sociedad Latinoamericana de Estimulacion Cardiaca y Electrofisiologia (SOLAECE)-Latin American Society of Cardiac Pacing and Electrophysiology. Endorsed by the American College of Cardiology (ACC) and American Heart Association (AHA). Europace 2015;18(2):159–83.

27. McAlister FA, Ezekowitz J, Hooton N, et al. Cardiac resynchronization therapy for patients with left ventricular systolic dysfunction: a systematic review. JAMA 2007;297(22):2502–14.

28. Wang S-B, Foster DB, Rucker J, et al. Redox regulation of mitochondrial ATP synthase: implications for cardiac resynchronization therapy. Circ Res 2011;109(7):750–7.

29. Agnetti G, Kaludercic N, Kane LA, et al. Modulation of mitochondrial proteome and improved mitochondrial function by biventricular pacing of dyssynchronous failing hearts. Circ Cardiovasc Genet 2010;3(1):78–87.

30. Aiba T, Hesketh GG, Barth AS, et al. Electrophysiological consequences of dyssynchronous heart failure and its restoration by resynchronization therapy. Circulation 2009;119(9):1220–30.

31. Chakir K, Daya SK, Aiba T, et al. Mechanisms of enhanced beta-adrenergic reserve from cardiac resynchronization therapy. Circulation 2009;119(9):1231–40.

32. Kass DA, Chen CH, Curry C, et al. Improved left ventricular mechanics from acute VDD pacing in patients with dilated cardiomyopathy and ventricular conduction delay. Circulation 1999;99(12):1567–73.

33. Cazeau S, Leclercq C, Lavergne T, et al. Effects of multisite biventricular pacing in patients with heart failure and intraventricular conduction delay. N Engl J Med 2001;344(12):873–80.

34. Cleland JGF, Daubert J-C, Erdmann E, et al. The effect of cardiac resynchronization on morbidity and mortality in heart failure. N Engl J Med 2005;352(15):1539–49.

35. Cleland JGF, Freemantle N, Daubert JC, et al. Long-term effect of cardiac resynchronisation in patients reporting mild symptoms of heart failure: a report from the CARE-HF study. Heart 2008;94(3):278–83.

36. Bristow MR, Saxon LA, Boehmer J, et al. Cardiac-resynchronization therapy with or without an implantable defibrillator in advanced chronic heart failure. N Engl J Med 2004;350(21):2140–50.

37. Auricchio A, Fantoni C, Regoli F, et al. Characterization of left ventricular activation in patients with heart failure and left bundle-branch block. Circulation 2004;109(9):1133–9.

38. Fantoni C, Kawabata M, Massaro R, et al. Right and left ventricular activation sequence in patients with heart failure and right bundle branch block: a detailed analysis using three-dimensional non-fluoroscopic electroanatomic mapping system. J Cardiovasc Electrophysiol 2005;16(2):112–9 [discussion:120–1].

39. Richman JL, Wolff L. Left bundle branch block masquerading as right bundle branch block. Am Heart J 1954;47(3):383–93.

40. Sipahi I, Chou JC, Hyden M, et al. Effect of QRS morphology on clinical event reduction with cardiac resynchronization therapy: meta-analysis of randomized controlled trials. Am Heart J 2012; 163(2):260–7.e3.

41. Chatterjee NA, Upadhyay GA, Singal G, et al. Precapillary pulmonary hypertension and right ventricular dilation predict clinical outcome in cardiac resynchronization therapy. JACC Heart Fail 2014; 2(3):230–7.

42. Derval N, Steendijk P, Gula LJ, et al. Optimizing hemodynamics in heart failure patients by systematic screening of left ventricular pacing sites: the lateral left ventricular wall and the coronary sinus are rarely the best sites. J Am Coll Cardiol 2010; 55(6):566–75.

43. Gold MR, Yu Y, Singh JP, et al. The effect of left ventricular electrical delay on AV optimization for cardiac resynchronization therapy. Heart Rhythm 2013;10(7):988–93.

44. Gold MR, Birgersdotter-Green U, Singh JP, et al. The relationship between ventricular electrical delay and left ventricular remodelling with cardiac resynchronization therapy. Eur Heart J 2011;32(20):2516–24.

45. Auricchio A, Delnoy P-P, Butter C, et al. Feasibility, safety, and short-term outcome of leadless ultrasound-based endocardial left ventricular resynchronization in heart failure patients: results of the wireless stimulation endocardially for CRT (WiSE-CRT) study. Europace 2014;16(5):681–8.

46. ALternate Site Cardiac ReSYNChronization (ALSYNC) Study. Available at: https://clinicaltrials.gov/show/NCT01277783. Accessed May 2, 2016.

47. Kamath GS, Balaram S, Choi A, et al. Long-term outcome of leads and patients following robotic epicardial left ventricular lead placement for cardiac resynchronization therapy. Pacing Clin Electrophysiol 2011;34(2):235–40.

48. Ellenbogen KA, Gold MR, Meyer TE, et al. Primary results from the SmartDelay determined AV optimization: a comparison to other AV delay methods used in cardiac resynchronization therapy (SMART-AV) trial: a randomized trial comparing empirical, echocardiography-guided, and algorithmic atrioventricular delay programming in cardiac resynchronization therapy. Circulation 2010; 122(25):2660–8.

49. Singh JP, Abraham WT, Chung ES, et al. Clinical response with adaptive CRT algorithm compared with CRT with echocardiography-optimized atrioventricular delay: a retrospective analysis of multicentre trials. Europace 2013;15(11):1622–8.

50. Abraham WT, Compton S, Haas G, et al. Intrathoracic impedance vs daily weight monitoring for predicting worsening heart failure events: results of the Fluid Accumulation Status Trial (FAST). Congest Heart Fail 2011;17(2):51–5.

51. Konstam MA. Home monitoring should be the central element in an effective program of heart failure disease management. Circulation 2012;125(6): 820–7.

52. Cleland JGF, Louis AA, Rigby AS, et al, TEN-HMS Investigators. Noninvasive home telemonitoring for patients with heart failure at high risk of recurrent admission and death: the Trans-European Network-Home-Care Management System (TEN-HMS) study. J Am Coll Cardiol 2005; 45(10):1654–64.

53. Rose EA, Gelijns AC, Moskowitz AJ, et al. Long-term use of a left ventricular assist device for end-stage heart failure. N Engl J Med 2001;345(20):1435–43.

54. Slaughter MS, Rogers JG, Milano CA, et al. Advanced heart failure treated with continuous-flow left ventricular assist device. N Engl J Med 2009; 361(23):2241–51.

55. Aaronson KD, Slaughter MS, Miller LW, et al. Use of an intrapericardial, continuous-flow, centrifugal pump in patients awaiting heart transplantation. Circulation 2012;125(25):3191–200.

56. Miller LW, Pagani FD, Russell SD, et al. Use of a continuous-flow device in patients awaiting heart transplantation. N Engl J Med 2007;357(9):885–96.

57. Pagani FD, Miller LW, Russell SD, et al. Extended mechanical circulatory support with a continuous-flow rotary left ventricular assist device. J Am Coll Cardiol 2009;54(4):312–21.

58. Lietz K, Long JW, Kfoury AG, et al. Outcomes of left ventricular assist device implantation as destination therapy in the post-REMATCH era: implications for patient selection. Circulation 2007;116(5):497–505.

59. Kirklin JK, Naftel DC, Kormos RL, et al. Second INTERMACS annual report: More than 1,000 primary left ventricular assist device implants. J Heart Lung Transplant 2010;29(1):1–10.

60. Stehlik J, Edwards LB, Kucheryavaya AY, et al. The registry of the international society for heart and lung transplantation: 29th official adult heart transplant report—2012. J Heart Lung Transplant 2012; 31(10):1052–64.

61. Kirklin JK, Naftel DC, Pagani FD, et al. Sixth INTERMACS annual report_ A 10,000-patient database. J Heart Lung Transplant 2014;33(6):555–64.

62. Garan AR, Levin AP, Topkara V, et al. Early postoperative ventricular arrhythmias in patients with

continuous-flow left ventricular assist devices. J Heart Lung Transplant 2015;34(12):1611–6.

63. Bedi M, Kormos R, Winowich S, et al. Ventricular arrhythmias during left ventricular assist device support. Am J Cardiol 2007;99(8):1151–3.

64. Cantillon DJ, Tarakji KG, Kumbhani DJ, et al. Improved survival among ventricular assist device recipients with a concomitant implantable cardioverter-defibrillator. Heart Rhythm 2010;7(4): 466–71.

65. Garan AR, Yuzefpolskaya M, Colombo PC, et al. Ventricular arrhythmias and implantable cardioverter-defibrillator therapy in patients with continuous-flow left ventricular assist devices: need for primary prevention? J Am Coll Cardiol 2013;61(25):2542–50.

66. Feldman D, Pamboukian SV, Teuteberg JJ, et al. The 2013 International Society for Heart and Lung Transplantation Guidelines for mechanical circulatory support: executive summary. J Heart Lung Transplant 2013;32(2):157–87.

67. Mozes A, DeNofrio D, Pham DT, et al. Inappropriate implantable cardioverter-defibrillator therapy due to electromagnetic interference in patient with a HeartWare HVAD left ventricular assist device. Heart Rhythm 2011;8(5):778–80.

68. Reported ICD Experience. Thoratec. Available at: http://www.thoratec.com/medical-professionals/reported-icd-experience.aspx. Accessed January 1, 2016.

69. Gopinathannair R, Birks EJ, Trivedi JR, et al. Impact of cardiac resynchronization therapy on clinical outcomes in patients with continuous-flow left ventricular assist devices. J Card Fail 2015;21(3): 226–32.

Home Inotropes and Other Palliative Care

Mahazarin Ginwalla, MD, MS

KEYWORDS

- Palliative care • Inotropes • Heart failure • Hospice • Deactivation

KEY POINTS

- Patients with American College of Cardiology/American Heart Association stage D heart failure have limited options beyond standard medical therapy including home inotropes, heart transplantation, mechanical circulatory support, or palliative care/hospice.
- Medical therapy for heart failure should be continued even when the patient is under palliative care, unless it is not tolerated or on patient/family request.
- For patients who are not candidates for advanced therapies, chronic continuous outpatient intravenous inotropic therapy may improve the patient's symptoms and overall quality of life and reduce hospitalizations, but they may accelerate mortality. The goals of therapy should be discussed in detail with the patient and caregivers.
- Pharmacologic therapy should be used judiciously to treat symptoms in advanced heart failure patients including use of oxygen, opioids, and diuretics to control symptoms of anxiety, dyspnea, and pain.
- Deactivation of devices such as defibrillators and mechanical circulatory support at end-of-life should occur in conjunction with the palliative care team for optimal patient and family support.

INTRODUCTION

With a growing number of patients who have heart failure, there is also a steady increase in the number of patients with advanced heart failure. End-stage heart failure is classified under the American College of Cardiology/American Heart Association (ACC/AHA) as stage D heart failure and is refractory to conventional heart failure therapy. These patients have limited options including home inotropes, cardiac transplantation, mechanical circulatory support, and palliative care/hospice.[1] Many patients may not be candidates for advanced therapies because of their age, comorbidities, or psychosocial factors. Other patients may choose not to avail of these advanced therapies. It is increasingly recognized that in addition to cancer, high-quality end-of-life care should be an integral part of care that is provided for those with other advancing chronic life-limiting conditions such as advanced heart failure.

Palliative care is an important modality in the management of patients who are not candidates for advanced therapies and for those patients who do not desire to avail of these options. Patients with advanced heart failure have a multitude of somatic symptoms including dyspnea, chest pain, palpitations, fatigue, and leg edema and psychiatric symptoms such as depression and anxiety. These symptoms are a result of volume overload, low cardiac output, renal failure, chronic angina, and arrhythmias. These symptoms are difficult to manage with conventional therapy in the end-stage heart failure patient and can benefit from the palliative care approach of management. The principles of palliative care may be assimilated

Disclosure Statement: The author has nothing to disclose.
Department of Cardiovascular Medicine, Harrington Heart & Vascular Institute, University Hospitals Case Medical Center, 11100 Euclid Avenue, Cleveland, OH 44106, USA
E-mail address: Mahazarin.Ginwalla@UHhospitals.org

Heart Failure Clin 12 (2016) 437–448
http://dx.doi.org/10.1016/j.hfc.2016.03.005
1551-7136/16/$ – see front matter © 2016 Elsevier Inc. All rights reserved.

heartfailure.theclinics.com

in the management of heart failure patients during the entire continuum of their illness.[2]

DEFINITION OF PALLIATIVE CARE

Palliative care is defined by the World Health Organization as "an approach that improves the quality of life of patients and their families facing the problem associated with life-threatening illness, through the prevention and relief of suffering by means of early identification and impeccable assessment and treatment of pain and other problems, physical, psychosocial and spiritual." Palliative care does not exclude conventional life-prolonging treatment and may be integrated into the care of the patient with advanced heart failure to optimize symptom management and quality of life.[3]

TIMING OF REFERRAL FOR PALLIATIVE CARE

Several studies found that palliative care and hospice are underutilized in advanced heart failure patients. In fact, some studies report that less than 10% of advanced heart failure patients are referred for palliative care.[4,5] All patients with advanced heart failure should be evaluated by their cardiologist for potential benefit from referral to palliative care, especially those who are undergoing advanced therapy options. One of the complex decisions for the heart failure specialist involves the timing of referral for palliative care. Heart failure patients often have episodes of decompensation followed by periods of improvement and stability. Identifying patients with advanced heart failure can be challenging, even when using different predictive tools and models. Clinical markers that are helpful to predict prognosis include worsening symptoms, recurrent hospitalizations, worsening markers on cardiopulmonary exercise tests, and laboratory tests like biomarkers. Predictive tools, including the Seattle Heart Failure model, and quality-of-life questionnaires, like the Kansas City Cardiomyopathy Questionnaire, are available, but at best these provide a likelihood of life expectancy. It is, therefore, up to the clinician to integrate the clinical evaluation with the prognostic tools to assess the patient's overall prognosis.

Referral for evaluation by the palliative care team can help improve advance care planning and improve the quality of care and decision making for the patient and his or her family. According to the 2013 ACC/AHA guidelines, "palliative and supportive care is effective for patients with symptomatic advanced heart failure to improve quality of life (Class 1B recommendation). Before hospital discharge, at the first postdischarge visit, and in subsequent follow-up visits, the need for palliative care and hospice should be addressed in all heart failure patients (Class I B recommendation)."[6]

In patients who are being considered for a left ventricular assist device (LVAD) implantation or cardiac transplantation, it is helpful for the patient to establish advance directives and goals of care before the procedure, in case of subsequent complications that render the patient unable to make decisions for himself. This shared decision making helps the patient's families understand the patient's wishes and improves awareness on the patient and physician aspect.

Before the LVAD implantation, the palliative care team can assist in establishing a preparedness plan that outlines the conditions under which he or she desires the device to be turned off.[7] Central to a palliative approach to patient care is the establishment of shared decision making among the patient, families and surrogates, and the medical team.[8]

As symptoms of advanced heart failure progress, patients and their families may decide to forego all life-prolonging care and transition to hospice care. Usually, these patients have less than 6 months to live. Advanced planning with a multidisciplinary care approach is important to provide essential support to the patients and their families.

PHARMACOLOGIC THERAPIES IN ADVANCED HEART FAILURE PATIENTS
Inotropes

Inotropes are medications that improve the contractility of the heart, and are used in patients with low cardiac output or evidence of end-organ dysfunction. These medications can also affect the heart rate, peripheral vascular resistance, and pulmonary pressures. Inotropes commonly used include milrinone, dobutamine, and dopamine. Digoxin is a weak oral inotrope. Levosimendan is only approved for use in Europe.

Chronic Home Inotropes

Chronic inotropes are usually used in patients with advanced heart failure for a variety of indications, including bridging to transplantation, before use of permanent mechanical support, or for palliation. The use of these medications has been associated with improved symptoms and reduced rehospitalizations. Although inotropes have been presumed to increase mortality in advanced heart failure patients because of a higher rate of ventricular arrhythmias,[9] the extent of this increase in mortality is not clear. This finding is a result of studies that show a higher proportion of cardiac arrests in advanced heart failure patients where asystole and pulseless electrical activity is the documented initial rhythm, with less than 25% of sudden cardiac deaths caused by ventricular fibrillation.[10–12] Hence, a detailed discussion with the patient and his family should be held before continuation of inotropes, especially for the long term to discuss potential risks and benefits (**Box 1**).[13,14]

A proposed central mechanism to the increase in malignant arrhythmias with inotrope use involves a chronic increase in intracellular Ca^{2+}, which contributes to altered gene expression and apoptosis.[15] Thus, long-term, continuous intravenous inotropic support as palliative therapy for symptom control may be considered in patients with stage D heart failure despite optimal medical and device therapy (Class IIb). However, these medications are not recommended for the routine management of acute decompensated heart failure (Class IIIb).[6] Oral inotropic agents for example, levosimendan, pimobendan, and vesnarinone, have not been found to improve outcomes.[13,16–18]

If chronic continuous inotropic therapy is used for palliative management, right heart catheterization is necessary in most circumstances to document a hemodynamic response. According to regulations of the Centers for Medicare and Medicaid Services, a 20% increase in cardiac index or a 20% decrease in pulmonary capillary wedge pressure is required for reimbursement. A patient already started on inotropes without a right heart catheterization before initiation would need cessation of the inotrope to document baseline hemodynamic parameters to compare with improved hemodynamics after reinitiation of inotrope.[19]

Other issues to consider and discuss with the patient include the infection risk involved with chronic indwelling intravenous catheters and availability of resources at home or in the community. It is recommended that the patient has 24-hour caregiver support to help change inotrope infusion bags and for dressing changes. It is usually not recommended that patients drive while taking home inotropes because of the risk of arrhythmias; however, some patients do return to being physically able to conduct their normal lives and may be able to drive short distances depending on their overall condition and mentation.

If the patient makes the transition to hospice care, there may be difficulties with financial coverage of the inotrope, as the daily infusion costs are greater than the Medicare payment associated with hospice care. Also, the intravenous inotrope may be misconstrued to be intended for extension of the patient's life, and the hospice agency may not agree to cover it. Thus, the inotrope often needs to be discontinued before discharge home or to a facility with hospice care, usually accompanied by accelerated narcotic titration.[3] It is important that the continuation of palliative inotropes not be regulated by the hospice agency but be determined by patient and caregiver choice.

The median survival of patients on chronic inotropic therapy has generally been limited and on the order of 3 to 6 months.[15,20,21] However, there are notable exceptions in clinical practice, as recently reported. Hashim and colleagues[22] published their single-center retrospective series of 197 patients, which reported a median survival of 18 months. However, median survival was short (eg, 9 months) for those patients in whom continuous inotropes were for palliation, with a 1-year actuarial survival rate of 48% and a 2-year actuarial survival rate of 38%. Importantly, not only did filling pressures and cardiac output improve, but patients felt better on inotropes after discharge.[22]

The reasons for the differences in outcomes between this study and previous work are not quite clear (**Table 1**). Pinney and Stevenson[23] elaborated several possible reasons. One can surmise that the improved survival in this report was the result of significant continued use of neurohormonal antagonists, including β-blockers, compared with prior studies. For instance, 72% of patients in the study were continued on β-blockers.[22] In contrast, Gorodeski and colleagues[24] reported a survival of 1 year in patients with chronic inotropic management, but only 19% of patients were on β-blockade. Another reason for the improved survival may be related

---

Box 1
Factors to consider in the selection of patients for home inotropes

Patient's wishes

Arrhythmogenic potential of inotropes

Presence of defibrillator and frequency of prior ventricular arrhythmias

Infection risk owing to indwelling catheters

Other ongoing issues in patient, such as end-organ failure, severe debilitation, altered mental status, severe depression

Overall physical condition of the patient

Availability of caregiver support

Availability of community and hospice resources

Table 1
Comparison of inotropes and mortality in previous and current era

| | Inotrope Use in Previous Era | | Inotrope Use in Current Era | |
	Hershberger et al[20]	Hauptman et al[21]	Gorodeski et al[24]	Hashim et al[22]
Inotrope used	Dobutamine or milrinone	Dobutamine or milrinone	50% dobutamine; 50% milrinone	15% dobutamine; 85% milrinone
Dose of Inotrope	Dobutamine: 6.8 ± 3.4 µg/kg/min Milrinone: 0.6 ± 0.3 µg/kg/min	Not reported	Dobutamine: 5.4 ± 2.5 µg/kg/min Milrinone: 0.4 ± 0.2 µg/kg/min	Dobutamine: 4.4 µg/kg/min Milrinone: 0.3 µg/kg/min
History of prior ventricular tachycardia (%)	Not reported	Not reported	Not reported	30
Prevalence of defibrillators (%)	14	Not reported	65	84
Use of neurohormonal antagonists while on inotropes:				
β-blockers (%)	Not reported	15	19	72
Angiotensin-converting enzyme inhibitors (%)	69	36	40	50
Angiotensin receptor blocker (%)	2	9.60	5	13
Aldosterone antagonists (%)	Not reported	Not reported	44–59	59
Median survival	3.4 mo	3–6 mo	9–18 mo	18 mo (9 mo for patients on inotropes solely for palliation)
6-mo survival (%)	26	57	45	60
1-y survival (%)	6	43	50	48
Survival according to inotrope used	Not reported	Not reported	No significant difference in adjusted mortality	Milrinone better than dobutamine (P<.01)
Hospitalizations after inotrope initiated	Equivalent pre- and postinotrope	Reduced	Reduced	Reduced

to inotropic doses used in the study. Milrinone was used on average at 0.3 µg/kg/min, and dobutamine at 4.4 µg/kg/min, compared with 0.6 µg/kg/min and 7 to 10 µg/kg/min, respectively, in previous studies with a worse survival. This study also had a higher number of defibrillators compared with prior studies, with less than 10% of patients who did not have a defibrillator. Seventeen percent of patients received at least 1 defibrillator shock.[23]

A recent consensus statement from the Heart Failure Society of America (**Box 2**) documented several criteria to be fulfilled before discharging patients on chronic home inotropic therapy. These include optimization of neurohormonal antagonists and diuretics, clear demonstration of symptomatic and hemodynamic improvement with failed weaning attempts, documentation of refusal of a heart transplant or LVAD or noncandidacy for these therapies, and a discussion with the patient that inotropes may not help and worsen survival.[25] It should also be clinically evident that the patient symptomatically feels better; many patients will not have any improvement in symptoms despite improvements in laboratory function, and the utility of home inotropic therapy in this situation is not clear.

<table>
<tr><td>

Box 2
Guidelines for management of patients on home inotropes

Maintain lowest dose of inotrope necessary in combination with optimal dose of oral vasodilator.

Consider continuation of oral β-blocker if patient is on milrinone if hemodynamically tolerated.

Continue mineralocorticoid antagonist and diuretic therapy.

Consider adding digoxin to regimen for additional inotropic benefit and heart rate modulation if renal and liver function acceptable.

Consider using milrinone over other inotropes because of its longer half-life.

Advise on warning signs of infection related to indwelling catheters.

Discuss with patient preference for turning off defibrillator.

Consider regular laboratory testing to guide overall management.

Consider close monitoring on an outpatient basis to determine need for adjusting inotrope dosage.

</td></tr>
</table>

Home Inotropic Selection

Home inotrope selection is based on the hemodynamic response of the inotrope and the need for a concomitant β-blocker. The following characteristics (**Table 2**) need to be considered before initiation of the inotrope.

Milrinone

Milrinone is a bipyridine and inhibits the phosphodiesterase-3 intracellular enzyme, thus preventing the degradation of cyclic adenosine monophosphate (cAMP) within the cell. Increased cAMP levels increase activation of protein kinase A, which, in turn, leads to more influx of calcium into the cell. This increase in intracellular calcium stimulates myocardial contractility. Milrinone also reduces peripheral vascular resistance and vasodilates pulmonary vasculature via cAMP, which may improve right ventricular function. Because of its vasodilator effect, milrinone may not be tolerated in vasoplegic patients, including patients with an active infection.[26]

Intravenous milrinone is cleared renally, has a longer half-life (2–4 hours) than other inotropic medications, and is particularly useful if adrenergic receptors are downregulated or desensitized in the setting of chronic heart failure, or after chronic β-agonist administration. Milrinone bypasses the β-adrenergic receptor, whereas the increase in cyclic adenosine monophosphate with dobutamine depends on ligand binding to the β-adrenergic receptor.[27] Tachyphylaxis is a known phenomenon with dobutamine but is less commonly observed with milrinone. Finally, the cost of milrinone is greater than that of dobutamine despite the availability of a generic formulation.[26]

Despite improvement in symptoms, milrinone has been shown to increase arrhythmias, overall mortality, and rehospitalizations in patients with advanced heart failure in several trials.[28] Of note, the Outcomes of Prospective Trial of Intravenous Milrinone for Exacerbations in Chronic Heart

Table 2
Inotropes in end-stage heart failure

	Mechanism	Increase in Intracellular Calcium	Dosage	Half-life
Milrinone	Phosphodiesterase inhibitor	Yes	0.125–0.75 μg/kg/min	2–4 h
Dobutamine	Adrenergic β1>β2>α1 receptor agonist	Yes	2–20 μg/kg/min	2 min
Dopamine	Adrenergic and dopaminergic agonist	Yes	0.5–2 μg/kg/min ↑ renal blood flow; 5–10 μg/kg/min ↑ cardiac output, 10–20 μg/kg/min ↑ systemic vascular resistance	1 min
Digoxin	Sodium-potassium (Na-K) pump inhibitor	Yes	0.125–0.25 mg/d	36–48 h if renal function normal
Levosimendan	Calcium sensitizer	No	0.05–0.2 μg/kg/min	1 h; 70–80 h for active metabolite

Failure (OPTIME-CHF) was a randomized trial in 951 patients with severe systolic dysfunction using milrinone versus placebo for 48 hours and followed up for 60 days. Milrinone was associated with hypotension and atrial arrhythmias without any significant difference in mortality or rehospitalization. A post hoc analysis found higher mortality and rehospitalization rates in patients with ischemic cardiomyopathy; no significant difference was noted in nonischemic cardiomyopathy patients.[29] The Acute Decompensated Heart Failure Registry (ADHERE) showed a higher in-hospital mortality rate in patients with acute decompensated heart failure on milrinone or dobutamine compared with nesiritide and nitroglycerin.[30] Increased 6-month mortality and more frequent hospitalizations were also seen in the Prospective Randomized Milrinone Survival Evaluation (PROMISE) trial, which enrolled 1088 patients with severe chronic heart failure and left ventricular dysfunction who were randomly assigned to milrinone or placebo.[13] This finding highlights the importance of using milrinone and dobutamine only in select patients.

Dobutamine

Dobutamine is a catecholamine with $\beta1$ and $\beta2$ adrenergic agonist activity, which improves myocardial contractility and decreases left ventricular end-diastolic pressure. Dobutamine may cause hypotension when initiated because of peripheral vasodilatation by its effect on $\beta2$ receptors and should be used with caution if the patient is hypotensive. Higher doses of dobutamine are not preferred in patients with myocardial ischemia, as it can increase myocardial oxygen demand and induce tachycardia. Dobutamine cannot be used along with β-blockers because of their opposing effects. The half-life of dobutamine is only a few minutes. Dobutamine can uncommonly cause a hypersensitivity reaction leading to eosinophilic myocarditis and peripheral eosinophilia.[31,32]

Dopamine

Dopamine is an endogenous catecholamine, and its effect is dose dependent. At lower doses of less than 3 μg/kg/min, dopamine leads to vasodilatation in the body vasculature including coronary and renal arteries. An intermediate dose of dopamine (3–10 μg/kg/min) increases inotropy and chronotropy and increases pulmonary capillary wedge pressure. At higher doses (10–20 μg/kg/min), α-receptor–mediated vasoconstriction occurs, which increases the afterload. Higher doses are more often used for hypotension.

The benefit of low-dose dopamine on renal function in patients with heart failure has not been conclusively shown.[33] Low-dose dopamine and low-dose nesiritide were studied in the Renal Optimization Strategies Evaluation in Acute Heart Failure (ROSE-AHF) trial in hospitalized patients with acute decompensated heart failure and acute renal failure; however, there was no statistically significant improvement in renal function or symptoms.[34]

Digoxin

Digoxin can improve hemodynamics and lower heart rates without reducing blood pressure. Digoxin has been shown to improve symptoms and reduce hospitalizations, but it does not have mortality benefit in patients with chronic systolic heart failure.[35] A level between 0.5 and 0.8 ng/mL is recommended, and levels greater than 1.2 ng/mL are associated with increased mortality rate. Currently, digoxin use in symptomatic patients with heart failure with reduced ejection fraction despite optimal medical therapy has a class IIA indication in the American College of Cardiology/American Heart Association 2013 Heart Failure Guidelines,[6] and a IIB indication in the European Society of Cardiology Heart Failure Guidelines.[36] However, because of its narrow therapeutic window, it is of limited benefit in patients with advanced heart failure who often have multiple dynamic comorbidities, for example, renal dysfunction, that exacerbate its toxicity.

Levosimendan

Levosimendan is a calcium sensitizing drug that can exert its inotropic effect by increasing the sensitivity of the cardiomyocyte to intracellular calcium by binding to troponin C. Achieving an inotropic effect without increasing intracellular calcium may reduce the risk of arrhythmias. It also leads to vasodilatation by opening adenosine-triphosphate–sensitive potassium channels in vascular smooth muscle causing their relaxation leading to reduction in preload and afterload.[37]

Several studies assessed the benefit of levosimendan in advanced heart failure. In the Randomized Study on Safety and Effectiveness of Levosimendan in Patients with Left Ventricular Failure after an Acute Myocardial Infarct (RUS-SLAN) trial, levosimendan decreased the risk of worsening heart failure and death, and it did not cause worsening ischemia or hypotension.[38] In the Levosimendan Infusion versus Dobutamine (LIDO) study, levosimendan showed lower mortality at 1 and 6 months compared with dobutamine in severe systolic heart failure patients.[39] However, the Randomized Multicenter Evaluation of Intravenous Levosimendan Efficacy (REVIVE-II) study showed increased arrhythmias and hypotension but improved symptoms in acute decompensated heart failure patients.[40] Levosimendan is approved for use in Europe; it does not have US Food and Drug Administration approval for use in the United States. The European Society of Cardiology Guidelines recommend the use of intravenous levosimendan in patients with acutely decompensated heart failure when there is suspicion that chronic β-blockade is worsening hypotension and lessening the responsiveness to vasopressor drugs (grade IIb recommendation, level C evidence).[36]

OTHER MEDICATIONS IN ADVANCED HEART FAILURE

Management of symptoms in stage D heart failure patients should be aimed at optimizing heart failure treatment and addressing specific symptoms, such as dyspnea and fatigue. Other symptoms commonly encountered in end-stage heart failure include pain, depression, anxiety, insomnia, and worsened cognitive function. Medications specifically targeting symptom relief, such as opioids for analgesia and dyspnea, and antidepressants for the relief of depression and anxiety, are endorsed in current guidelines.[6] Nonsteroidal anti-inflammatory drugs should be avoided because of the high risks of gastrointestinal bleeding, renal failure, and fluid retention.[41]

Fluid overload should be reduced with diuretics, and fluid and salt intake should be restricted as tolerated to improve dyspnea and fatigue. Torsemide and bumetanide have better bioavailability and are preferred in advanced heart failure patients especially with refractory volume overload. Intravenous diuretics are needed for patients with a poor response to oral diuretic therapy. Angiotensin-converting enzyme inhibitors, angiotensin receptor blockers, β-blockers, hydralazine, nitrates, and aldosterone antagonists generally prolong survival and alleviate symptoms, and thus should not necessarily be discontinued in advanced disease. However, their role in extending longevity in end-stage advanced heart failure is not well established. Therefore, they may be discontinued if there are signs of hemodynamic stability, worsening end-organ function, or poor oral intake.[8]

NONPHARMACOLOGIC AND INVASIVE THERAPIES IN PALLIATIVE CARE

Patients with advanced heart failure on inotropic support who are candidates for cardiac resynchronization therapy (CRT) have anecdotally been rescued by this therapy. However, this strategy is controversial, as the clinical trials of device therapy excluded patients on inotropes, and patients requiring inotrope therapy had increased hospital mortality after device implantation in one study.[42] However, in some patients with positive clinical and electrocardiographic findings who have a high likelihood of responding to CRT, device implantation may be performed to attempt weaning off inotrope therapy.[43]

Additional device-related therapies that may help alleviate symptoms in the advanced heart failure patient include pacing at a higher rate, usually in the 70s to 80s at rest, to augment cardiac output. Chronic right ventricular pacing induces left ventricular dyssynchrony with deleterious effects on left ventricular function. However, short term right ventricular pacing may help improve symptoms of fatigue and shortness of breath in the advanced heart failure patient. Similarly in patients with CRT, increasing the rate of CRT pacing may help improve symptoms.[44]

Other invasive therapies for symptom improvement in advanced heart failure patients include indwelling pleural and peritoneal catheters for refractory or recurrent nonmalignant pleural effusions and ascites.[45] Palliative hemodialysis in the advanced palliative care patient may be continued if the patient is chronically dialysis dependent and wishes to continue hemodialysis for symptom management, although this is usually limited by hemodynamic difficulties with volume removal and does not improve the overall quality of life. Peritoneal dialysis may be a better option than hemodialysis in refractory heart failure patients because of its better hemodynamic tolerance and convenience.[46] Hemodialysis for acute renal failure in the end-stage heart failure patient is not recommended.

PALLIATIVE MEDICINE IN PATIENTS WITH LEFT VENTRICULAR ASSIST DEVICES

The LVAD is used in patients with advanced ACC/AHA stage D heart failure to improve quality of life, functional capacity, and survival.[47] The LVAD was originally developed as a bridge to transplant (BTT) for patients with advanced heart failure who decompensated while awaiting a heart transplant. LVAD is now also being used as destination therapy (DT) in patients who are not candidates for heart transplantation. This nomenclature is somewhat dynamic, as patients who have an LVAD as DT may become candidates for a heart transplant (eg, after smoking cessation), and, conversely, BTT LVAD patients may have an adverse event, such as cancer or stroke, and become DT LVAD patients.[48]

Although patients often experience significant improvement in some of their symptoms after

LVAD implantation, many other symptoms, including physical pain, major depression, adjustment disorders, and organic mental syndromes, may remain or occur de novo after VAD implantation. Patients may require repeated hospitalizations because of LVAD-related infections, strokes, and gastrointestinal bleeding. Given the complexity of decision making related to LVAD implantation, Thompson and colleagues[49] developed a Patient Decision Aid, which addresses a spectrum of cognitive and emotional aspects of end-of-life decision making and is helpful for the patient and caregiver before a DT LVAD implant. The advantage of early and longitudinal palliative care in these patients is the support provided with the changes in patient attitudes on experiencing the reality of living with the LVAD. Patients may require significantly more support from caregivers, and, in turn, caregiver fatigue is well recognized because of the increased burden of taking care of the LVAD patient. Therefore, palliative care may need to be continued or initiated after VAD placement to help the patient and support caregivers.

The 2013 ACC/AHA heart failure guidelines suggests that clinicians should address symptom control, psychological distress, health-related quality of life, patient preferences, and caregiver support, while providing ongoing access to evidence-based optimal medical therapy.[6] Addition of a palliative care member to the core interdisciplinary LVAD team has now been included as a requirement for Joint Commission Mechanical Circulatory Support certification.[50]

Patients undergoing BTT and DT LVAD implantation often have undefined goals of care and undocumented advance directives. Also, discussions regarding end-of-life care including withdrawal of device support may not be conducted; hence, ethical dilemmas may arise if the patient is terminal.[7] To avoid these situations in which the patient's wishes are unclear, it is important to consult palliative medicine to address end-of-life preferences and facilitate advance care planning. This consultation is also termed *preparedness planning*, which is consistent with the patients' goals and specifically addresses circumstances in the event the patient has an adverse outcome. This planning includes decisions regarding appointment of a patient surrogate decision maker and patient care preferences in the event of poor quality of life, acute device failure, catastrophic complications like a stroke, or a progressive comorbid condition such as renal failure or cancer. These advance directives provide physicians, patient families, and surrogates insight into the patients' health care goals and preferences, and

ease the decision-making process at the time of withdrawal of mechanical circulatory support.[7,47]

Patients may have acute VAD dysfunction or develop complications or progression of comorbid conditions.[8] The management of VAD patients near the end of life poses unique challenges to the patient, family, and care providers, and active participation of the palliative care team is important when LVAD deactivation is considered. The palliative care team can help provide valuable assistance to ensure that the patient's symptoms are controlled when MCS is discontinued and to provide additional assistance in supporting the patient's family.

DEACTIVATION OF PACEMAKERS AND DEFIBRILLATORS IN END-STAGE HEART DISEASE

Patients with advanced heart failure commonly have cardiovascular implantable electronic devices (CIED), which include pacemaker (PM), defibrillator (ICD), and CRT devices. Requests to deactivate CIEDs occur because patients may reach a point at which the therapies delivered are no longer helpful but are a burden and not consistent with their health care wishes. Advance care planning including advance directives and living will should include a discussion of these patient preferences. The shared decision-making approach in which clinicians and the palliative care team work together with the patients and families is particularly helpful to ensure that patients understand the burdens of a particular therapy and the potential outcomes of its discontinuation. For patients with advanced heart failure in palliative care, it is reasonable to forego replacing the generator of a CIED with the patient's consent if it is at end of life.

The withdrawal of the CIED function must be understood in the context of its particular function. The PM is indicated for bradycardia and not only does it have life-prolonging function in patients who are pacemaker dependent, but it is also indicated for symptom control such as dizziness. In a pacemaker-dependent patient, death will follow immediately after terminating PM therapy. A CRT device is indicated for improvement of symptoms owing to heart failure, and its discontinuation may also impact survival as well as symptoms and quality of life of the end-stage heart failure patient. However, as ICDs are implanted for prevention of sudden death in patients at risk, deactivation of ICD shock therapy may improve quality of life, as it will avoid ICD discharges, which are more likely to occur as heart failure worsens. Multiple options are available regarding the extent of deactivation of the CIED, including selective deactivation of only the shock therapy and continuation of the pacing feature of the PM and CRT device.[51] Data suggest that most patients or surrogates (79% in one study) who request CIED deactivation are those who want to avoid shocks during the dying process.[52] Patients on chronic inotropes may also decide to have their ICD shock therapy deactivated, and this is an important discussion that should occur before the patient's discharge on home inotropes. Patients may have symptoms including pain, dyspnea, and anxiety related to device deactivation. Preparations should be made before deactivation of the device to ensure that their symptoms are appropriately managed.

HOSPICE CARE

As patients with advanced heart failure have progression of their disease, they may decide to forego all life-prolonging care and transition to hospice care. Eligibility for nonhospice palliative care is based on patient needs and does not depend on prognosis. In comparison, hospice provides palliative care for the dying patient who has a prognosis less than 6 months and does not want any treatments aimed at curing their primary illness.[53] In cases in which the patient has been referred to hospice, the hospice benefit provides continued grief and bereavement counseling for the family for up to 1 year after the patient's death.[54]

Despite the benefits of organized hospice care at end-of-life, the referral of advanced heart failure patients to hospice is underutilized.[4,55] In 2006, it was estimated that 11% of patients who died of advanced heart failure were enrolled in hospice programs. Reasons for underutilization are proposed to be uncertain prognosis/disease course, increasing number of available therapies, lack of clinical evidence to support palliative care and hospice care, and inadequate training.[56] Encouraging, however, are data that show that there was an apparent increase in use over the last decade. Medicare beneficiary data from patients with the specific diagnosis of HF from 2000 to 2007 show a significant increase in hospice services, with nearly 40% these beneficiaries using hospice services in the most recent years evaluated.[57]

Hospice data suggest that advance directives specifying limitations in end-of-life care are associated with significantly lower levels of Medicare spending, lower likelihood of in-hospital death, and higher use of hospice care in regions characterized by higher levels of end-of-life spending.[58]

There are data to suggest that Medicare beneficiaries with heart failure who received hospice had an increased mean survival of 81 days compared with those heart failure patients who did not receive hospice.[59] With interdisciplinary collaboration between heart failure cardiologists and palliative care teams, patients dying under hospice care may have improved satisfaction with the dying process in their preferred place of care.

FUTURE DIRECTIONS

Over the last few years, the advent of new pharmacologic and innovative device therapies has altered the facade of advanced heart failure dramatically. A key challenge is the recognition of the severity of heart failure, and the determination of utility versus futility given the patient's clinical condition and comorbidities. There is a growing population of advanced heart failure patients who are not candidates for these therapies or choose not to avail of them. This group benefits from integration of their health care with palliative care or transitioning to hospice to improve quality of life, improve symptoms, and allow continuity of health care services.

SUMMARY POINTS

1. Patients with ACC/AHA stage D heart failure have progressed to the point that their options include heart transplant, mechanical support, home inotropes, experimental protocols, or palliative care/hospice.
2. The focus of palliative care is symptom relief but does not preclude reasonable active treatment unless the patient has transitioned to hospice. Medical therapy for heart failure should be continued unless it is not tolerated or at the request of the patient/family.
3. Hauptman PJ. Heart failure: Palliative Care in end- stage heart disease. Adult Clinical Cardiology Self-Assessment Self- Assessment Program Book set (ACCSAP 8) 2012;11(12):1–5.
4. Continuous intravenous inotrope therapy may be considered for patients who are not candidates for cardiac transplant or ventricular assist device therapy but requires significant caregiver support.
5. Inotropes may improve the patient's symptoms and overall quality of life but may accelerate mortality. The goals of therapy should be discussed in detail with the patient and caregivers.
6. Several different inotrope options are available. The optimal inotrope dose in combination with oral vasodilators should be

determined by hemodynamic tailored therapy before discharging the patient on home inotropes.

7. β-blockade should be continued if tolerated by patients on home milrinone.

8. Judicious use of oxygen, opioids, and diuretics should be used to control symptoms of anxiety, dyspnea, and pain.

9. Unlike defibrillators, CRT is found to improve quality of life. Therefore, it may be appropriate to continue biventricular pacing for patients even when the decision has been made to turn off ICDs.

10. In patients who are being considered for an LVAD implantation, it is critical that the patient establishes advance directives before implantation and has a preparedness plan that outlines the conditions under which he or she desires the device to be turned off.

11. Selective deactivation of an ICD should be discussed with the patient and family members when the patient enters the terminal phase of heart failure to prevent shocks in a dying patient.

12. Hospice care is a specialized form of palliative care in which the patient has decided to forgo all life-prolonging treatment. Hospice patients usually have a life expectancy of less than 6 months.

REFERENCES

1. Hunt SA, Baker DW, Chin MH, et al. ACC/AHA guidelines for the evaluation and management of chronic heart failure in the adult: executive summary a report of the American College of Cardiology/American Heart Association task force on practice guidelines (committee to revise the 1995 guidelines for the evaluation and management of heart failure): developed in collaboration with the international society for heart and lung transplantation; endorsed by the heart failure society of America. Circulation 2001;104:2996–3007.

2. Hauptman PJ, Havranek EP. Integrating palliative care into heart failure care. Arch Intern Med 2005; 165:374–8.

3. Hauptman PJ. Heart failure: palliative care in end-stage heart disease. 2012.

4. Greener DT, Quill T, Amir O, et al. Palliative care referral among patients hospitalized with advanced heart failure. J Palliat Med 2014;17:1115–20.

5. Kavalieratos D, Mitchell EM, Carey TS, et al. "Not the 'grim reaper service'": an assessment of provider knowledge, attitudes, and perceptions regarding palliative care referral barriers in heart failure. J Am Heart Assoc 2014;3:e000544.

6. Yancy CW, Jessup M, Bozkurt B, et al. 2013 ACCF/AHA guideline for the management of heart failure: a report of the American College of Cardiology Foundation/American Heart Association task force on practice guidelines. J Am Coll Cardiol 2013;62:e147–239.

7. Swetz KM, Freeman MR, AbouEzzeddine OF, et al. Palliative medicine consultation for preparedness planning in patients receiving left ventricular assist devices as destination therapy. Mayo Clin Proc 2011;86:493–500.

8. Adler ED, Goldfinger JZ, Kalman J, et al. Palliative care in the treatment of advanced heart failure. Circulation 2009;120:2597–606.

9. Acharya D, Sanam K, Revilla-Martinez M, et al. Infections, arrhythmias, and hospitalizations on home intravenous inotropic therapy. Am J Cardiol 2016; 117(6):952–6.

10. Tung P, Albert CM. Causes and prevention of sudden cardiac death in the elderly. Nat Rev Cardiol 2013;10:135–42.

11. Youngquist ST, Kaji AH, Niemann JT. Beta-blocker use and the changing epidemiology of out-of-hospital cardiac arrest rhythms. Resuscitation 2008;76:376–80.

12. Teodorescu C, Reinier K, Uy-Evanado A, et al. Survival advantage from ventricular fibrillation and pulseless electrical activity in women compared to men: the Oregon Sudden Unexpected Death Study. J Interv Card Electrophysiol 2012;34:219–25.

13. Packer M, Carver JR, Rodeheffer RJ, et al. Effect of oral milrinone on mortality in severe chronic heart failure. The PROMISE Study Research Group. N Engl J Med 1991;325:1468–75.

14. Felker GM, O'Connor CM. Inotropic therapy for heart failure: an evidence-based approach. Am Heart J 2001;142:393–401.

15. Stevenson LW. Clinical use of inotropic therapy for heart failure: looking backward or forward? part II: chronic inotropic therapy. Circulation 2003;108:492–7.

16. Cohn JN, Goldstein SO, Greenberg BH, et al. A dose-dependent increase in mortality with vesnarinone among patients with severe heart failure. Vesnarinone Trial Investigators. N Engl J Med 1998;339:1810–6.

17. Jalanko M, Kivikko M, Harjola VP, et al. Oral levosimendan improves filling pressure and systolic function during long-term treatment. Scand Cardiovasc J 2011;45:91–7.

18. Koizumi T, Taguchi S. Low-dose oral pimobendan emancipates patients with severe ischemic pump failure from intravenous catecholamine infusion for cardiogenic shock. Int J Cardiol 2016;202:829–30.

19. CGS Administrators L. Durable medical equipment regional carrier. Available at: http://www.cgsmedicare.com/jc/pubs/adv/pdf/1995/December%201995.pdf.

Centers for Medicare and medicaid services. Home parenteral inotropic therapy: data collection form. Available at: https://coverage.cms.fu.com/lcd_area/lcd_uploads/5044_15/HomeParenterallnotropic-Therapy DataCollectionForm.pdf. Accessed September 29, 2011.

20. Hershberger RE, Nauman D, Walker TL, et al. Care processes and clinical outcomes of continuous outpatient support with inotropes (COSI) in patients with refractory endstage heart failure. J Card Fail 2003;9:180–7.

21. Hauptman PJ, Mikolajczak P, George A, et al. Chronic inotropic therapy in end-stage heart failure. Am Heart J 2006;152:1096.e1–8.

22. Hashim T, Sanam K, Revilla-Martinez M, et al. Clinical characteristics and outcomes of intravenous inotropic therapy in advanced heart failure. Circ Heart Fail 2015;8:880–6.

23. Pinney SP, Stevenson LW. Chronic inotropic therapy in the current era: old wines with new pairings. Circ Heart Fail 2015;8:843–6.

24. Gorodeski EZ, Chu EC, Reese JR, et al. Prognosis on chronic dobutamine or milrinone infusions for stage D heart failure. Circ Heart Fail 2009;2:320–4.

25. Fang JC, Ewald GA, Allen LA, et al. Advanced (stage D) heart failure: a statement from the Heart Failure Society of America Guidelines Committee. J Card Fail 2015;21:519–34.

26. Colucci WS, Wright RF, Jaski BE, et al. Milrinone and dobutamine in severe heart failure: differing hemodynamic effects and individual patient responsiveness. Circulation 1986;73:III175–83.

27. Lowes BD, Tsvetkova T, Eichhorn EJ, et al. Milrinone versus dobutamine in heart failure subjects treated chronically with carvedilol. Int J Cardiol 2001;81: 141–9.

28. Amsallem E, Kasparian C, Haddour G, et al. Phosphodiesterase III inhibitors for heart failure. Cochrane Database Syst Rev 2005;(1):CD002230.

29. Felker GM, Benza RL, Chandler AB, et al. Heart failure etiology and response to milrinone in decompensated heart failure: results from the OPTIME-CHF study. J Am Coll Cardiol 2003;41:997–1003.

30. Abraham WT, Adams KF, Fonarow GC, et al. In-hospital mortality in patients with acute decompensated heart failure requiring intravenous vasoactive medications: an analysis from the acute decompensated heart failure national registry (ADHERE). J Am Coll Cardiol 2005;46:57–64.

31. Takkenberg JJ, Czer LS, Fishbein MC, et al. Eosinophilic myocarditis in patients awaiting heart transplantation. Crit Care Med 2004;32:714–21.

32. El-Sayed OM, Abdelfattah RR, Barcelona R, et al. Dobutamine-induced eosinophilia. Am J Cardiol 2004;93:1078–9.

33. Bellomo R, Chapman M, Finfer S, et al. Low-dose dopamine in patients with early renal dysfunction: a placebo-controlled randomised trial. Australian and New Zealand Intensive Care Society (ANZICS) Clinical Trials Group. Lancet 2000;356:2139–43.

34. Chen HH, Anstrom KJ, Givertz MM, et al. Low-dose dopamine or low-dose nesiritide in acute heart failure with renal dysfunction: the ROSE acute heart failure randomized trial. JAMA 2013;310:2533–43.

35. Digitalis Investigation Group. The effect of digoxin on mortality and morbidity in patients with heart failure. N Engl J Med 1997;336:525–33.

36. McMurray JJ, Adamopoulos S, Anker SD, et al. ESC guidelines for the diagnosis and treatment of acute and chronic heart failure 2012: the task force for the diagnosis and treatment of acute and chronic heart failure 2012 of the European Society of Cardiology. Developed in collaboration with the Heart Failure Association (HFA) of the ESC. Eur J Heart Fail 2012;14:803–69.

37. Tariq S, Aronow WS. Use of inotropic agents in treatment of systolic heart failure. Int J Mol Sci 2015;16: 29060–8.

38. Moiseyev VS, Poder P, Andrejevs N, et al. Safety and efficacy of a novel calcium sensitizer, levosimendan, in patients with left ventricular failure due to an acute myocardial infarction. A randomized, placebo-controlled, double-blind study (RUSSLAN). Eur Heart J 2002;23:1422–32.

39. Follath F, Cleland JG, Just H, et al. Efficacy and safety of intravenous levosimendan compared with dobutamine in severe low-output heart failure (the LIDO study): a randomised double-blind trial. Lancet 2002;360:196–202.

40. Packer M, Colucci W, Fisher L, et al. Effect of levosimendan on the short-term clinical course of patients with acutely decompensated heart failure. JACC Heart Fail 2013;1:103–11.

41. Qaseem A, Snow V, Shekelle P, et al. Evidence-based interventions to improve the palliative care of pain, dyspnea, and depression at the end of life: a clinical practice guideline from the American College of Physicians. Ann Intern Med 2008;148: 141–6.

42. Swindle J, Burroughs TE, Schnitzler MA, et al. Short-term mortality and cost associated with cardiac device implantation in patients hospitalized with heart failure. Am Heart J 2008;156:322–8.

43. Braunschweig F, Hauptman PJ. Cardiac resynchronization therapy in the intensive care setting; the promise and peril of using implantable devices off label. Eur J Heart Fail 2008;10:220–1.

44. Vardas PE, Auricchio A, Blanc JJ, et al. Guidelines for cardiac pacing and cardiac resynchronization therapy: the task force for cardiac pacing and cardiac resynchronization therapy of the European Society of Cardiology. Developed in collaboration with the European Heart Rhythm Association. Eur Heart J 2007;28:2256–95.

45. Herlihy JP, Loyalka P, Gnananandh J, et al. PleurX catheter for the management of refractory pleural effusions in congestive heart failure. Tex Heart Inst J 2009;36:38–43.

46. Lu R, Mucino-Bermejo MJ, Ribeiro LC, et al. Peritoneal dialysis in patients with refractory congestive heart failure: a systematic review. Cardiorenal Med 2015;5:145–56.

47. Rose EA, Gelijns AC, Moskowitz AJ, et al. Long-term use of a left ventricular assist device for end-stage heart failure. N Engl J Med 2001;345:1435–43.

48. Teuteberg JJ, Stewart GC, Jessup M, et al. Implant strategies change over time and impact outcomes: insights from the INTERMACS (interagency registry for mechanically assisted circulatory support). JACC Heart Fail 2013;1:369–78.

49. Thompson JS, Matlock DD, McIlvennan CK, et al. Development of a decision aid for patients with advanced heart failure considering a destination therapy left ventricular assist device. JACC Heart Fail 2015;3:965–76.

50. Joint Commission Disease-Specific Certification Program. Advanced certification heart failure performance implementation measurement guide; Revisions to requirements for advanced certification for VAD, Effective March 23, 2014. Certification Manual.

51. Lampert R, Hayes DL, Annas GJ, et al. HRS expert consensus statement on the management of cardiovascular implantable electronic devices (CIEDs) in patients nearing end of life or requesting withdrawal of therapy. Heart Rhythm 2010;7:1008–26.

52. Buchhalter LC, Ottenberg AL, Webster TL, et al. Features and outcomes of patients who underwent cardiac device deactivation. JAMA Intern Med 2014;174:80–5.

53. Morrison RS, Meier DE. Clinical practice. Palliative care. N Engl J Med 2004;350:2582–90.

54. Goldstein NE, May CW, Meier DE. Comprehensive care for mechanical circulatory support: a new frontier for synergy with palliative care. Circ Heart Fail 2011;4:519–27.

55. Cheung WY, Schaefer K, May CW, et al. Enrollment and events of hospice patients with heart failure vs. cancer. J Pain Symptom Manage 2013;45:552–60.

56. Berry JI. Hospice and heart disease: missed opportunities. J Pain Palliat Care Pharmacother 2010;24:23–6.

57. Unroe KT, Greiner MA, Johnson KS, et al. Racial differences in hospice use and patterns of care after enrollment in hospice among Medicare beneficiaries with heart failure. Am Heart J 2012;163:987–93.e3.

58. Nicholas LH, Langa KM, Iwashyna TJ, et al. Regional variation in the association between advance directives and end-of-life Medicare expenditures. JAMA 2011;306:1447–53.

59. Connor SR, Pyenson B, Fitch K, et al. Comparing hospice and nonhospice patient survival among patients who die within a three-year window. J Pain Symptom Manage 2007;33:238–46.

Recovery Versus Remission: Clinical Insights

Peter C. Ferrin, BA[a,1], Lauren McCreath, BA[a,1], Sutip Navankasattusas, PhD[b],
Stavros G. Drakos, MD, PhD[a,c,1,*]

KEYWORDS

- Heart failure • Cardiomyopathy • Recovery • Remission • Reverse remodeling

KEY POINTS

- In advanced chronic heart failure, reverse remodeling leads to better long-term outcomes and improved, but usually not completely normalized, myocardial function and biology.
- The recovered chronic heart failure population still experiences significant rates of heart failure–related adverse events.
- Especially for chronic advanced heart failure the term *remission* may be more appropriate than *recovery*. Although complete durable recovery has been seen in acute and subacute presentations of heart failure, it has yet to be shown at a meaningful scale in chronic advanced heart failure.
- As heart failure therapies evolve and populations of patients who experience reverse myocardial remodeling grow, insights from clinical and translational studies will guide us in bridging remission and true recovery.

INTRODUCTION

Medical, surgical, and device therapies reverse pathologic remodeling that occurs in heart failure (HF), which leads to decreased morbidity and mortality. Many acute dilated cardiomyopathies recover significant endogenous cardiac function spontaneously, whereas reverse remodeling in advanced chronic HF is typically only achieved by medical intervention. HF patients have traditionally been classified into 1 of 2 groups based on their left ventricular (LV) ejection fraction (EF)—HF with preserved EF (HFpEF; EF >50%) or HF with reduced EF (HFrEF; EF <50%). However, with the current abundance of therapies that result in substantial reverse myocardial remodeling in a significant proportion of patients across etiologies, a third group is emerging. This group consists of patients who previously had a reduced EF, but responded well to current HF therapies and improved their EF to greater than 50%. Patients from this third group, generally referred to as *HF recovered*, seem clinically similar to HFpEF patients, but the groups are pathologically distinct, and the HF-recovered patients have better event-free survival compared with their HFpEF and HFrEF counterparts.[1] In this review, we focus on the clinical and molecular factors that underlie the processes and maintenance of myocardial recovery.

Cardiac remodeling that leads to systolic HF in part comprises compensatory mechanisms the

Disclosures: The authors have no relationships to disclose.
[a] Molecular Medicine Program, University of Utah, 15 North 2030 East, Salt Lake City, UT 84112, USA;
[b] Division of Cardiovascular Medicine, University of Utah School of Medicine, Molecular Medicine Program, Eccles Institute of Human Genetics and UTAH Cardiac Transplant Program, Salt Lake City, Utah, USA; [c] Utah Transplantation Affiliated Hospitals (UTAH) Cardiac Transplant Program, University of Utah Health Sciences Center, Intermountain Medical Center, Veterans Affairs Salt Lake City Health Care System, 50 Medical Drive, Salt Lake City, UT 84132, USA
[1] These authors contributed equally to this article.
* Corresponding author. Division of Cardiovascular Medicine, University of Utah, 15 North 2030 East, Room 4420, Salt Lake City, UT.
E-mail address: stavros.drakos@hsc.utah.edu

Heart Failure Clin 12 (2016) 449–459
http://dx.doi.org/10.1016/j.hfc.2016.03.007

heart uses in an attempt to overcome the disease process. What is initially an attempt to heal eventually becomes overcompensatory, causing maladaptive hypertrophy, wall thinning, and a decreased stroke volume characteristic of HFrEF.[2,3] Molecular changes underlie the macroscopic increase in size and rounding of the heart's ventricles. These changes include cardiomyocyte hypertrophy, increased cell death, changes in excitation contraction coupling, β-adrenergic desensitization, changes in collagen content and organization, decreased microvascular density, and abnormal energetics characterized by decreased mitochondrial capacity and altered substrate utilization.[2–4] Many aspects of this complex cardiac remodeling process have been well characterized.[2–4]

Reverse myocardial remodeling is the process by which many of the harmful adaptations that occur during cardiac remodeling are inverted. This process can occur across a variety of clinical settings and disease severities, although it occurs to different extents in different patients depending on the specific cause of disease; each individual responds differently. A large percentage of acute dilated cardiomyopathy patients often undergo spontaneous and rapid reverse remodeling once the initial insult is alleviated.[5] Medical, surgical, and device therapies can also prompt reverse remodeling by correcting many of the harmful cellular changes that occur in cardiac remodeling but usually not all of them. Reverse remodeling is not an all-or-none phenomenon, nor is it necessarily long lasting. However, most successful therapies that result in clinical benefits involve some degree of reverse remodeling. The molecular and clinical processes that accompany reverse myocardial remodeling for a variety of treatments have been described.[6–8]

It is important to distinguish between myocardial recovery and remission. HF patients with reduced EF theoretically follow 1 of 3 trajectories:

1. Progression of disease: despite therapy, the patient's EF remains low or worsens, cardiac remodeling pathologic abnormalities remain, and long-term prognosis is poor.
2. Remission: the heart initially responds to treatment and improves clinically and biologically, but the HF condition eventually recurs, because of either the original insult or a new one.
3. Recovery: the heart responds to treatment and recovers, expressing normalized biology, and the condition can be considered cured.

Recovery from HF implies sustained improvement with normalized function, structure, and biology, whereas *remission* can be defined as a degree of improvement accompanied by incomplete biological normalization, reduced but not ameliorated HF hospitalizations, and HF recurrence (**Fig. 1**).[1] Although complete durable recovery has been seen in acute and subacute presentations of HF, it has yet to be seen at a meaningful rate in chronic advanced HF.

POTENTIAL FOR RECOVERY IN RECENT-ONSET CARDIOMYOPATHIES

Patients with recent-onset cardiomyopathies (ROCM) caused by abnormal energetics, toxins, and inflammation are more likely to recover when compared with those with chronic sustained HF.[9] Improvement often occurs even in the absence of disease-modifying therapies, and for those that do require therapies, recovery potential is high.

The populations that recover spontaneously generally have sustained long-term recovery, indicating that the process of recovering from these acute and subacute insults may be more a true normalization of heart function than reverse remodeling that results from surgical, device, or medical therapies in chronic HF patients.[5,10] In some cases, this recovery includes complete normalization of protein expression, a process that is usually not seen in the chronic HF recovered population but is seen in recovered Takotsubo cardiomyopathy patients.[11] This finding may be because in a rapid-onset disease mechanism the cells do not have time to increase in size; there is not a sustained period for significant reorganization of extracellular matrix and collagen deposition. The acute immune response of ROCM leads to different signaling and activation of different pathways than the immune response of chronic HF. However, this theory is just speculation—there is currently little evidence to prove this theory. The rate and nature of spontaneous recovery from various acute causes are listed in **Table 1**. However, improvement rates vary widely, particularly across certain demographic groups. For example, black patients have significantly lower EF improvement at 6 months than nonblacks[9]; black women with peripartum cardiomyopathy had more LV dysfunction at 6 and 12 months postpartum.[12]

Although observation of spontaneous recovery from acute and subacute HF finds remarkable myocardial plasticity and potential to recover from significant myocardial defects, studies in this area have not provided a thorough understanding of the underlying molecular mechanisms of recovery.[6] Of note, patients who are younger and have shorter durations of symptoms (less

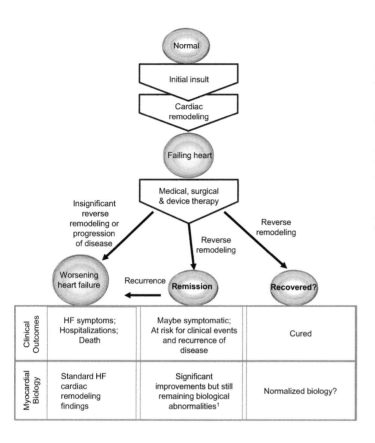

Fig. 1. Significant reverse remodeling of the failing heart results in remission or recovery. *Remission* is a state of incomplete recovery in which function, biology, and outcomes are partially improved, but HF recurs. *Recovery* is a state of complete functional improvement and biological normalization. Although true recovery is observed at significant rates for recent onset cardiomyopathies, complete functional and biological recovery from chronic HF has not been seen at significant rates, even after medical, surgical, and device therapies.

than 3–6 months) are more likely to improve their function and structure.[13]

POTENTIAL FOR CLINICAL AND MOLECULAR RECOVERY IN CHRONIC HEART FAILURE ETIOLOGIES

The rate and timing of significant reverse remodeling seen in chronic HF etiologies is compared with those of acute and subacute etiologies in **Table 1**.

Drug Therapies

Neurohormonal blockade is the cornerstone of HF management and improves clinically relevant outcomes, including death and HF hospitalizations.[14] These drugs slow the progression of HF, and β-blockers and renin-angiotensin-aldosterone system (RAAS) antagonists are also associated with significant reverse remodeling.

β-adrenergic blockers
Although many large randomized trials found improved long-term survival for HF patients on β-blockers, the MERIT-HF (Metoprolol CR/XL Randomised Intervention Trial in Congestive Heart Failure) trial and RESOLVD (Randomized evaluation of strategies for left ventricular dysfunction)

pilot study found that treatment with metoprolol for 6 months actually led to decreased LV chamber volumes and increased LVEF. Carvedilol elicits a similar response.[15,16] The REVERT (REversal of VEntricular Remodeling with Toprol-XL) trial found that metoprolol's reverse remodeling effect was most evident in patients with mild LV dilation and no advanced HF symptoms.

β-blockers are found to reverse some of the molecular dysfunction of the failing heart, including reversal of the fetal gene program. Patients with idiopathic dilated cardiomyopathy who had an improved EF with β-blockade also had increased sarcoplasmic-reticulum calcium ATPase and α-myosin heavy-chain mRNA expression and decreased β-myosin heavy chain mRNA expression, although expression of genes related to β-adrenergic receptors remained unchanged.[17] The fact that β-blockers contribute to the reversal of the maladaptive fetal gene expression seen in HF is important because reverse remodeling often does not normalize the failing heart gene expression. The current molecular signatures of improved HF are more suggestive of a condition in remission rather than truly recovered, which should be indistinguishable from normal healthy hearts.

Table 1
Myocardial recovery in various HF populations

Disease Etiology of HF	Therapies Tested	Responder Rate[a]	Timing to Response	Durability of Response[b]
Alcoholic cardiomyopathy[5,58]	Alleviation of toxic insult	Not well defined because of differences in alcohol consumption, estimated at 40%–80%	Months to years	Strong
Chemotherapy-induced cardiomyopathy[5]	Alleviation of toxic insult	70%–80%	<6 mo	Medium/strong?
Hemodynamic overload (mitral and aortic valve abnormalities)[59–61]	β-blockade, RAAS antagonism, aortic valve replacement, mitral valve replacement/repair	~25%	Months–1 y	Varied[c]
Chronic idiopathic dilated cardiomyopathy[14,52,62]	β-blockade, RAAS antagonism, VAD, resynchronization	20%–80%	3–6 mo	?
Chronic ischemic cardiomyopathy[14,63,64]	β-blockade, RAAS antagonism, VAD, revascularization, resynchronization	20%–60%	3–6 mo	?
Myocarditis[5,65]	Azathioprine and cyclosporine or azathioprine and prednisone, VAD	40%–100%	Days to months	Strong/medium?
Peripartum cardiomyopathy[5,66]	Bromocriptine, pentoxifylline, cardiac support device	60%–100%	Within 6 mo	Medium/strong?
Systemic inflammatory response syndrome[5]	Alleviation of sepsis	60%–100%	7–10 d	Strong
Tachycardia-induced cardiomyopathy[5,67]	Management varies depending on arrhythmia type	80%–90%	3–6 mo	Medium/strong
Takotsubo cardiomyopathy[5,68]	Diuretics, vasodilators, β-blockade	90%–100%	Weeks–1 y	Strong
Thyroid disease[5,69]	Treatment of underlying thyroid disease	~90%	3 mo	Strong

? The fact that the durability of response for these etiologies is currently not well defined.

[a] Defined as significant improvement of function, as most trials examined both improvements in myocardial function and clinical outcomes.

[b] Lack of good-quality, quantifiable data regarding the durability of response for many of these etiologies; this area represents a major unmet need in contemporary HF clinical management and research.

[c] Although there is evidence that mitral valve replacement/repair leads to reverse remodeling, there is debate as to whether this reverse remodeling actually leads to improved survival.

Renin-angiotensin-aldosterone system antagonism

Antagonism of the RAAS by angiotensin-converting enzyme (ACE) inhibitors, angiotensin receptor blockers, and aldosterone antagonists is found to retard cardiac remodeling and, to a lesser extent, even promote reverse remodeling.[18–21] Small-scale studies indicate that dual antagonism of the RAAS by the combination of the aldosterone antagonist, spironolactone, and the angiotensin antagonist, candesartan, further reduced LV chamber volumes while increasing EF.[22] RAAS antagonism also improves some of the structural abnormalities associated with systolic HF. Failing hearts have higher-than-normal collagen content, which increases wall stress and wall stiffness.[23] A study of the cellular effects of ACE inhibitors showed the treated group had decreased myocardial fibrosis compared with patients not taking ACE inhibitors.[24]

Surgical Therapies

Mitral valve replacement and repair

Amelioration of mitral regurgitation can lead to reverse remodeling and improved EF, but patients who relapse into HF after mitral valve repair or replacement do so with concomitant adverse cardiac remodeling and recurrent mitral regurgitation.[25] Yet, it is unclear whether mitral valve replacement or repair actually leads to improved morbidity and mortality. For patients with severe ischemic mitral valve regurgitation, there are no significant differences in survival or adverse events between those who undergo valve replacement and those who undergo repair, but those who underwent replacement had less recurrence of mitral regurgitation.[26]

Aortic valve replacement

Aortic stenosis represents the quintessential pressure overload model of HF, and aortic valve replacement can lead to dramatic resolution of LV function and decrease in LV size. In a recent study, patients who underwent aortic valve replacement had maximum LV mass regression by 24 months for patients with aortic stenosis, whereas regression plateaued at nearly 5 years for patients with aortic regurgitation. In addition, LV recovery after this procedure was correlated with better survival and freedom from HF.[27]

Revascularization

For a subset of HF patients with chronic HF as a result of an ischemic insult, medical and surgical/catheter-based revascularization leads to reverse remodeling and improvement of HF symptoms.[6] LV function often improves substantially after revascularization as stunned or hibernating myocardium regains contractility.[6] Fibrosis content and the extent of molecular remodeling affect the time course and possible extent of recovery, but, in the absence of scar, delayed recovery of hibernating myocardium is possible and may even stimulate myocyte proliferation.[28] Surgical reshaping of the ventricle in addition to revascularization initially showed further promise. However, the STICH (The Surgical Treatment for Ischemic Heart Failure) trial found no differences in exercise tolerance, hospitalizations, or mortality between groups that received both revascularization and ventriculoplasty compared with just revascularization, despite greater decreases in LV end-systolic volume for the group who received both treatments.[29]

Device Therapies

Cardiac resynchronization therapy

For HF patients with a wide QRS complex, cardiac resynchronization therapy (CRT) leads to regression of ventricular hypertrophy and increased EF across a wide spectrum of HF classes.[30] On a molecular level, CRT is associated with changes in the regional heterogeneity in left ventricular gene expression, shifts the expression of key mitochondrial proteins that normalize Krebs cycle intermediates, improves cardiomyocyte contractility and calcium handling by upregulating β-1 receptors, suppresses G_1-coupled signaling, and reduces subcellular heterogeneity of t-tubules.[31,32] On a functional level, CRT resynchronizes the ventricles, improves atrioventricular synchronization, and shifts the LV pressure-volume relationship to the left.[31]

CRT results in significant myocardial recovery in two-thirds of patients as defined by a decrease in end systolic volume and an increase in EF. CRT super-responders are also described when the resulting EF is greater than 50%. Being female, having no prior myocardial infarction, QRS duration greater than 150 ms, left bundle branch block, body mass index less than 30 kg/m, and smaller baseline left atrial volume index are all strong indicators of a super-response.[33,34] For those that recover EF, the recovery seems to be durable. The longest follow-up of any CRT trial was the MADIT-CRT (The Multicenter Automatic Defibrillator Implantation Trial – Cardiac Resynchronization Therapy) trial, which found that after 2.4 years the favorable changes induced by CRT remained.

VENTRICULAR ASSIST DEVICES: THE EMERGING FIELD OF UNLOADING-INDUCED RECOVERY/REMISSION FOR ADVANCED HEART FAILURE PATIENTS

Mechanical unloading-induced recovery is emerging as a potential outcome for a subset of advanced HF. It has long been observed that implantation of left ventricular assist devices (LVADs) often leads to varying degrees of reverse remodeling. LVADs, both pulsatile- and continuous-flow, alleviate stress on the myocardium by reducing the hemodynamic overload that drives the vicious cycle of myocardial dysfunction. LVADs are typically reserved for patients with advanced HF who are either waiting for transplant (bridge to transplant) or are ineligible for transplant (the so called destination therapy). In a subset of advanced HF patients, the LVAD-induced reverse remodeling and associated cardiac recovery is significant enough to consider device explantation.[10,35,36] Functional improvement seems to occur more frequently in patients with a nonischemic cardiomyopathy,[37-40] although selected ischemic cardiomyopathy patients also show a propensity to improve.[41] As is the case in ROCM, younger LVAD patients and patients with shorter durations of symptomatic HF are more likely to improve.[42]

LVAD use also provides a major asset for researchers—cardiac tissue can be obtained from the left ventricular apex at the time of device implant, and at the time of transplant or explant, resulting in paired tissue samples that can document the structural-, cellular-, and molecular-level aspects of the reverse remodeling process. In addition, because of lack of available donor organs and improving device performance, there is now a fairly large population of HF patients with LVADs. The relatively small subpopulation of LVAD patients who recover after device implantation provide unique insight into the pathology of the failing and recovered heart both because their tissue is available at multiple time points and because the level of illness is so advanced. The insight gained from examining the tissue of these patients can be projected onto the broader HF population and may suggest new therapies that target phylogenetically conserved pathways involved directly in myocardial recovery.

Mechanical unloading normalizes or reverses many of the harmful biological processes of HF. The enlarged cardiomyocytes, characteristic of hypertrophic cardiomyopathy, regress in size although not to the point of disuse atrophy.[43] Contractile defects are reversed as a result of improved Ca^{2+} handling and normalization of cytoskeletal protein expression. β–adrenergic signaling improves as a result of recovered β-adrenergic receptor density and distribution. Cell death is reduced. Pulsatile and continuous-flow LVADs also increase microvascular density despite the depleted state of HF.[10,23] Other factors are partially normalized by circulatory support. The levels of key neurohormones change after unloading, although not in a uniform manner.[44] Investigations have found conflicting results of LVAD unloading's effect on extracellular matrix composition and organization—some studies found a decrease in collagen content and others found an increase.[44] Additionally, the extent of remodeling owing to unloading varies from patient to patient, and the effects of the LVAD are often indistinguishable from the impact of simultaneous drug administration.[10]

In general, prospective studies have reported much higher rates of functional improvement than retrospective studies, with prospective studies explanting between 10% and 60% of patients (**Fig. 2**).[37-40,45-52] The difference in observed recovery rates between prospective and retrospective studies may be because of lack of serial assessment of LV function after device implant, lack of specific guidelines for antiremodeling drug regimen, lack of standardized criteria for LVAD explantation in retrospective studies, variability in the degree of unloading, and pulsatility dictated by pump speed; surgical technique and clinical setting variation may also influence these outcomes. The highest rates of recovery are observed when an aggressive adjuvant HF drug protocol is administered to the enrolled patients. Administration of the β2–agonist, clenbuterol, in addition to β1-blockers, ACE inhibitors, and aldosterone antagonists, led to sufficient recovery of LV function to allow pulsatile LVAD explantation in rates higher than 60%.[38,40] These observations were extended in a study of continuous-flow LVADs, in which 63% of patients recovered enough function to justify LVAD explantation.[39] Importantly, these studies were small and without a control group. The addition of clenbuterol to the typical HF pharmacologic therapies may have played a role in the high incidence of reverse remodeling in these small-scale LVAD studies, but the evidence remains sparse. Importantly, the sustainability of these improved responses remains unclear. Freedom from HF recurrence or death was 88.9% 4 years after explantation and 83.3% 3 years after explantation in these pulsatile-flow and continuous-flow studies.[38,39]

A critical clinical step for the LVAD-induced recovery field will be to determine the durability of recovery after device explantation. Most centers with sufficient experience with LVAD facilitated

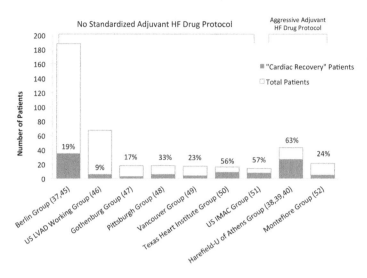

Fig. 2. Rates of functional improvement to the point of VAD explant in prospective unloading-induced recovery studies. *Cardiac recovery* is defined as device explantation because of myocardial improvement. Results from both of the Harefield studies[38,39] and the University of Athens study[40] were combined because they used the same bridge-to-recovery protocol. US IMAC, US intervention in myocarditis and acute cardiomyopathy. (*Adapted from* Drakos SG, Mehra MR. Clinical myocardial recovery during long-term mechanical support in advanced heart failure: insights into moving the field forward. J Heart Lung Transplant 2016;35(4):413–20; with permission.)

myocardial recovery do see relapse of HF in explanted patients, although some patients may have prolonged stability. However, the relapse rate is unclear, with freedom from HF recurrence after explant varying from 20% to 100% in different studies with follow-up times ranging from 6 months to 8 years.[10] In a large study of 53 explanted patients monitored for 5 years after device explant, one-third eventually had HF recurrence. Pre-explant echocardiographic parameters were found to be strongly correlated with recurrence.[44] Another large-scale study compared the clinical trajectory of patients who were explanted with a control group of HF patients who received transplants. Interestingly, those who were explanted showed comparable survival, lower secondary failure rates, and lower rates of longer-term complications than the patients who received transplants.[53] In the case of idiopathic cardiomyopathy, if the initial insult remains unresolved at the time of explant, the patient is likely to experience postexplant worsening of cardiac function. Although most recovery studies have not monitored their explanted patients for long periods, the North American RESTAGE-HF (Remission From Stage D Heart Failure) trial that has recently completed its enrolment of 40 patients will monitor the explanted patients for a prolonged period to better understand the durability of LVAD-induced recovery.

SUSTAINED RECOVERY

Accurately predicting who will benefit from different therapies resulting in sustained long-term improvement is a major contemporary research focus.[54] Younger patients and patients with a short duration of HF show greater propensity to recover function with improved biology than older patients with long histories of ventricular dysfunction.[37,39,42] This finding is hypothesized by some to be related to cardiac plasticity.[6] Like a balloon, the heart is predicted to be elastic to a point and can expand while still being able to structurally reverse. However, once the hypertrophy surpasses a point-of-no-return, the elastic deformation may switch to plastic deformation, from which the heart cannot recover.

Because chronic HF-recovered patients are generally younger with shorter duration of HF, a case can be made that invasive therapies like LVAD implantation should begin to be implemented earlier if medical therapies are not slowing or reversing the disease progression. The ROADMAP (Risk Assessment and Comparative Effectiveness of Left Ventricular Assist Device and Medical Management) study compared patients who opted for early LVAD implantation with their counterparts who elected to continue with pharmacologic therapy.[55] This study found that there is not a mortality case for early LVAD implantation—there were twice as many adverse events in the LVAD group as there were in the medical group—but those who chose early implantation had significantly reduced depression and increased quality of life.[55] This finding may be significant, as patient-centered factors might also be associated with myocardial biologic improvement or deterioration and, as a result, recovery and remission in a bidirectional way.

Although younger patients with shorter duration of HF are overrepresented in the HF-recovered population, these metrics do not hold a great amount of quantifiable predictive value for who will or will not recover and whose recovery will be sustainable.

An important first step in determining recoverability could be an evaluation of myocardial potential to recover through identification of dysfunctional but viable myocardium using advanced imaging modalities.[56] Combined with molecular biomarkers and traditional methods of evaluating function, such as echocardiography, this type of advanced phenotyping may prove beneficial in identifying those with the highest potential to respond given the heterogeneous and unpredictable nature of the broad advanced HF population.

There is currently little evidence for predictive biomarkers that can accurately forecast who will respond to different therapies and who has the potential for sustained recovery. However, biomarkers may provide a biological signature of HF remission and recovery.[1] Biomarker-guided HF therapy also shows promise in optimizing the efficacy and durability of response of HF therapies. By adjusting therapies based on suppression/normalization of biomarkers rather than symptoms and structural metrics, recovery may be more effectively achieved. Brain natriuretic peptide (BNP) and N-terminal pro-brain natriuretic peptide (NT-proBNP) have shown the best results in guiding therapy,[57] but development of a robust, multimarker guidance strategy could be even more effective. Although the results of preliminary studies are encouraging, large outcomes-based trials are needed to develop such a biomarker panel and prove the superiority of biomarker-guided HF therapy. Ideally, biomarkers with low biological, statistical, and analytical variability will be identified to help distinguish recovery versus remission patients and guide treatments. These treatments could then be incorporated with clinical and molecular data to create a risk score for sustainable myocardial recovery.

SUMMARY

The difference between remission and recovery in chronic HF patients is not well understood. Future studies focused on patient groups with significant reverse remodeling and recovery of function need to effectively correlate functional and biological/molecular data and include in their study design long-term follow-up to distinguish recovery from remission.

Understanding the biological processes that allow failing hearts with low EF to recover substantial function should be a primary goal of HF research. It is also important to determine which factors play a role regarding whether an improved heart maintains its recovered EF or is in remission and regresses back to a state of reduced EF. Finally, it is critical to determine which factors are still abnormal in the state of remission, and how to normalize those factors, in order for recovering hearts to fully heal.

REFERENCES

1. Basuray A, French B, Ky B, et al. Heart failure with recovered ejection fraction: clinical description, biomarkers, and outcomes. Circulation 2014;129: 2380–7.
2. Cohn JN, Ferrari R, Sharpe N. Cardiac remodeling–concepts and clinical implications: a consensus paper from an international forum on cardiac remodeling. Behalf of an International Forum on Cardiac Remodeling. J Am Coll Cardiol 2000;35: 569–82.
3. Mann DL. Mechanisms and models in heart failure: a combinatorial approach. Circulation 1999;100: 999–1008.
4. Mann DL, Barger PM, Burkhoff D. Myocardial and the failing heart: myth, magic, or molecular target? J Am Coll Cardiol 2012;60:2465–72.
5. Givertz MM, Mann DL. Epidemiology and natural history of recovery of left ventricular function in recent onset dilated cardiomyopathies. Curr Heart Fail Rep 2013;10:321–30.
6. Hellawell JL, Margulies KB. Myocardial reverse remodeling. Cardiovasc Ther 2012;30:172–81.
7. Kramer DG, Trikalinos TA, Kent DM, et al. Quantitative evaluation of drug or device effects on ventricular remodeling as predictors of therapeutic effects on mortality in patients with heart failure and reduced ejection fraction: a meta-analytic approach. J Am Coll Cardiol 2010;56:392–406.
8. Koitabashi N, Kass DA. Reverse remodeling in heart failure–mechanisms and therapeutic opportunities. Nat Rev Cardiol 2012;9:147–57.
9. McNamara DM, Starling RC, Cooper LT, et al. Clinical and demographic predictors of outcomes in recent onset dilated cardiomyopathy: results of the IMAC (intervention in myocarditis and acute cardiomyopathy)-2 study. J Am Coll Cardiol 2011; 58:1112–8.
10. Drakos SG, Kfoury AG, Stehlik J, et al. Bridge to recovery: understanding the disconnect between clinical and biological outcomes. Circulation 2012;126: 230–41.
11. Wittstein IS, Thiemann DR, Lima JA, et al. Neurohumoral features of myocardial stunning due to sudden emotional stress. N Engl J Med 2005; 352:539–48.
12. McNamara DM, Elkayam U, Alharethi R, et al, IPAC Investigators. Clinical outcomes for peripartum cardiomyopathy in North America: results of the IPAC

study (investigations of pregnancy-associated cardiomyopathy). J Am Coll Cardiol 2015;66:905–14.

13. Steimle AE, Stevenson LW, Fonarow GC, et al. Prediction of improvement in recent onset cardiomyopathy after referral for heart transplantation. J Am Coll Cardiol 1994;23:553–9.

14. Yancy CW, Jessup M, Bozkurt B, et al. 2013 ACCF/AHA guideline for the management of heart failure: executive summary: a report of the American College of Cardiology Foundation/American Heart Association Task Force on practice guidelines. Circulation 2013;128:1810–52.

15. Torp-Pedersen C, Poole-Wilson PA, Swedberg K, et al, COMET Investigators. Effects of metoprolol and carvedilol on cause-specific mortality and morbidity in patients with chronic heart failure–COMET. Am Heart J 2005;149:370–6.

16. Packer M, Antonopoulos GV, Berlin JA, et al. Comparative effects of carvedilol and metoprolol on left ventricular ejection fraction in heart failure: results of a meta-analysis. Am Heart J 2001;141:899–907.

17. Lowes BD, Gilbert EM, Abraham WT, et al. Myocardial gene expression in dilated cardiomyopathy treated with beta-blocking agents. N Engl J Med 2002;346:1357–65.

18. St John Sutton M, Lee D, Rouleau JL, et al. Left ventricular remodeling and ventricular arrhythmias after myocardial infarction. Circulation 2003;107:2577–82.

19. Danser AH, van Kesteren CA, Bax WA, et al. Prorenin, renin, angiotensinogen, and angiotensin-converting enzyme in normal and failing human hearts. Evidence for renin binding. Circulation 1997;96:220–6.

20. Wong M, Staszewsky L, Latini R, et al, Val-HeFT Heart Failure Trial Investigators. Valsartan benefits left ventricular structure and function in heart failure: Val-HeFT echocardiographic study. J Am Coll Cardiol 2002;40:970–5.

21. Greenberg B, Quinones MA, Koilpillai C, et al. Effects of long-term enalapril therapy on cardiac structure and function in patients with left ventricular dysfunction. Results of the SOLVD echocardiography substudy. Circulation 1995;91:2573–81.

22. Chan AK, Sanderson JE, Wang T, et al. Aldosterone receptor antagonism induces reverse remodeling when added to angiotensin receptor blockade in chronic heart failure. J Am Coll Cardiol 2007;50:591–6.

23. Drakos SG, Kfoury AG, Hammond EH, et al. Impact of mechanical unloading on microvasculature and associated central remodeling features of the failing human heart. J Am Coll Cardiol 2010;56:382–91.

24. Klotz S, Burkhoff D, Garrelds IM, et al. The impact of left ventricular assist device-induced left ventricular unloading on the myocardial renin-angiotensin-aldosterone system: therapeutic consequences? Eur Heart J 2009;30:805–12.

25. Hung J, Papakostas L, Tahta SA, et al. Mechanism of recurrent ischemic mitral regurgitation after annuloplasty: continued LV remodeling as a moving target. Circulation 2004;110:II85–90.

26. Goldstein D, Moskowitz AJ, Gelijns AC, et al, CTSN. Two-year outcomes of surgical treatment of severe ischemic mitral regurgitation. N Engl J Med 2016;374:344–53.

27. Une D, Mesana L, Chan V, et al. Clinical impact of changes in left ventricular function after aortic valve replacement: analysis from 3112 patients. Circulation 2015;132:741–7.

28. Page BJ, Banas MD, Suzuki G, et al. Revascularization of chronic hibernating myocardium stimulates myocyte proliferation and partially reverses chronic adaptations to ischemia. J Am Coll Cardiol 2015;65:684–97.

29. Jones RH, Velazquez EJ, Michler RE, et al, STICH Hypothesis 2 Investigators. Coronary bypass surgery with or without surgical ventricular reconstruction. N Engl J Med 2009;360:1705–17.

30. Ukkonen H, Beanlands RS, Burwash IG, et al. Effect of cardiac resynchronization on myocardial efficiency and regional oxidative metabolism. Circulation 2003;107:28–31.

31. Leyva F, Nisam S, Auricchio A. 20 years of cardiac resynchronization therapy. J Am Coll Cardiol 2014;64:1047–58.

32. Li H, Lichter JG, Seidel T, et al. Cardiac resynchronization therapy reduces subcellular heterogeneity of ryanodine receptors, T-Tubules, and Ca2+ sparks produced by dyssynchronous heart failure. Circ Heart Fail 2015;8:1105–14.

33. Hsu JC, Solomon SD, Bourgoun M, et al, MADIT-CRT Executive Committee. Predictors of super-response to cardiac resynchronization therapy and associated improvement in clinical outcome: the MADIT-CRT (multicenter automatic defibrillator implantation trial with cardiac resynchronization therapy) study. J Am Coll Cardiol 2012;59:2366–73.

34. Proclemer A, Muser D, Facchin D. What we can learn from "Super-responders". Card Electrophysiol Clin 2015;7:781–8.

35. Drakos SG, Mehra MR. Clinical myocardial recovery during long-term mechanical support in advanced heart failure: insights into moving the field forward. J Heart Lung Transplant 2016. http://dx.doi.org/10.1016/j.healun.2016.01.001.

36. Selzman CH, Madden JL, Healy AH, et al. Bridge to removal: a paradigm shift for left ventricular assist device therapy. Ann Thorac Surg 2015;99:360–7.

37. Dandel M, Weng Y, Siniawski H, et al. Heart failure reversal by ventricular unloading in patients with chronic cardiomyopathy: criteria for weaning from

ventricular assist devices. Eur Heart J 2011;32: 1148–60.

38. Birks EJ, Tansley PD, Hardy J, et al. Left ventricular assist device and drug therapy for the reversal of heart failure. N Engl J Med 2006;355:1873–84.

39. Birks EJ, George RS, Hedger M, et al. Reversal of severe heart failure with a continuous-flow left ventricular assist device and pharmacological therapy: a prospective study. Circulation 2011; 123:381–90.

40. Drakos SG, Terrovitis JV, Anastasiou-Nana MI, et al. Reverse remodeling during long-term mechanical unloading of the left ventricle. J Mol Cell Cardiol 2007;43:231–42.

41. Wever-Pinzon J, Al-Sarie M, Catino A, et al. Structural and functional myocardial improvement following continuous-flow mechanical unloading in chronic ischemic and non-ischemic cardiomyopathy [abstract]. J Heart Lung Transplant 2015;34:S126–7.

42. Goldstein DJ, Maybaum S, MacGillivray TE, et al, HeartMate II Clinical Investigators. Young patients with nonischemic cardiomyopathy have higher likelihood of left ventricular recovery during left ventricular assist device support. J Card Fail 2012;18: 392–5.

43. Diakos NA, Selzman CH, Sachse FB, et al. Myocardial atrophy and chronic mechanical unloading of the failing human heart: implications for cardiac assist device-induced myocardial recovery. J Am Coll Cardiol 2014;64:1602–12.

44. Dandel M, Weng Y, Siniawski H, et al. Pre-explant stability of unloading-promoted cardiac improvement predicts outcome after weaning from ventricular assist devices. Circulation 2012; 126:S9–19.

45. Dandel M, Weng Y, Siniawski H, et al. Prediction of cardiac stability after weaning from left ventricular assist devices in patients with idiopathic dilated cardiomyopathy. Circulation 2008;118:S94–105.

46. Maybaum S, Mancini D, Xydas S, et al. Cardiac improvement during mechanical circulatory support: a prospective multicenter study of the LVAD Working Group. Circulation 2007;115:2497–505.

47. Liden H, Karason K, Bergh CH, et al. The feasibility of left ventricular mechanical support as a bridge to cardiac recovery. Eur J Heart Fail 2007;9:525–30.

48. Gorcsan J 3rd, Severyn D, Murali S, et al. Non-invasive assessment of myocardial recovery on chronic left ventricular assist device: results associated with successful device removal. J Heart Lung Transplant 2003;22:1304–13.

49. Lamarche Y, Kearns M, Josan K, et al. Successful weaning and explantation of the Heartmate II left ventricular assist device. Can J Cardiol 2011;27: 358–62.

50. Khan T, Delgado RM, Radovancevic B, et al. Dobutamine stress echocardiography predicts myocardial improvement in patients supported by left ventricular assist devices (LVADs): hemodynamic and histologic evidence of improvement before LVAD explantation. J Heart Lung Transplant 2003;22: 137–46.

51. Boehmer JP, Starling RC, Cooper LT, et al, IMAC Investigators. Left ventricular assist device support and myocardial recovery in recent onset cardiomyopathy. J Card Fail 2012;18:755–61.

52. Patel SR, Saeed O, Murthy S, et al. Combining neurohormonal blockade with continuous-flow left ventricular assist device support for myocardial recovery: a single-arm prospective study. J Heart Lung Transplant 2013;32:305–12.

53. Birks EJ, George RS, Firouzi A, et al. Long-term outcomes of patients bridged to recovery versus patients bridged to transplantation. J Thorac Cardiovasc Surg 2012;144:190–6.

54. Bonios MJ, Wever-Pinzon J, Stehlik J, et al. Cardiac rotational mechanics as a predictor of favorable functional and structural response after mechanical unloading with cardiac assist devices in advanced heart failure patients. HFSA new investigator award finalist abstract. J Card Fail 2015;21:S4.

55. Estep JD, Starling RC, Horstmanshof DA, et al, ROADMAP Study Investigators. Risk assessment and comparative effectiveness of left ventricular assist device and medical management in ambulatory heart failure patients: results from the ROADMAP study. J Am Coll Cardiol 2015;66: 1747–61.

56. Wilcox JE, Fonarow GC, Ardehali H, et al. "Targeting the Heart" in heart failure: myocardial recovery in heart failure with reduced ejection fraction. JACC Heart Fail 2015;3:661–9.

57. Januzzi JL, Troughton R. Are serial BNP measurements useful in heart failure management? Serial natriuretic peptide measurements are useful in heart failure management. Circulation 2013;127:500–7 [discussion: 508].

58. Guzzo-Merello G, Segovia J, Dominguez F, et al. Natural history and prognostic factors in alcoholic cardiomyopathy. JACC Heart Fail 2015; 3:78–86.

59. Geidel S, Lass M, Schneider C, et al. Downsizing of the mitral valve and coronary revascularization in severe ischemic mitral regurgitation results in reverse left ventricular and left atrial remodeling. Eur J Cardiothorac Surg 2005;27:1011–6.

60. Magalhaes MA, Koifman E, Torguson R, et al. Outcome of left-sided cardiac remodeling in severe aortic stenosis patients undergoing transcatheter aortic valve implantation. Am J Cardiol 2015;116: 595–603.

61. Westenberg JJ, Braun J, Van de Veire NR, et al. Magnetic resonance imaging assessment of reverse left ventricular remodeling late after restrictive mitral annuloplasty in early stages of dilated cardiomyopathy. J Thorac Cardiovasc Surg 2008;135:1247–52 [discussion: 1252–3].

62. Drakos SG, Wever-Pinzon O, Selzman CH, et al, UCAR (Utah Cardiac Recovery Program) Investigators. Magnitude and time course of changes induced by continuous-flow left ventricular assist device unloading in chronic heart failure: insights into cardiac recovery. J Am Coll Cardiol 2013;61:1985–94.

63. Bodi V, Monmeneu JV, Ortiz-Perez JT, et al. Prediction of reverse remodeling at cardiac MR imaging soon after first ST-segment-elevation myocardial infarction: results of a large prospective registry. Radiology 2016;278:54–63.

64. Morishita T, Uzui H, Mitsuke Y, et al. Predictive utility of the changes in matrix metalloproteinase-2 in the early phase for left ventricular reverse remodeling after an acute myocardial infarction. J Am Heart Assoc 2015;4:e001359.

65. Mason JW, O'Connell JB, Herskowitz A, et al. A clinical trial of immunosuppressive therapy for myocarditis. The Myocarditis Treatment Trial Investigators. N Engl J Med 1995;333:269–75.

66. Desplantie O, Tremblay-Gravel M, Avram R, et al, BRO-HF Initiative Investigators. The medical treatment of new-onset peripartum cardiomyopathy: a systematic review of prospective studies. Can J Cardiol 2015;31:1421–6.

67. Medi C, Kalman JM, Haqqani H, et al. Tachycardia-mediated cardiomyopathy secondary to focal atrial tachycardia: long-term outcome after catheter ablation. J Am Coll Cardiol 2009; 53:1791–7.

68. Sharkey SW, Maron BJ. Epidemiology and clinical profile of takotsubo cardiomyopathy. Circ J 2014; 78:2119–28.

69. Siu CW, Yeung CY, Lau CP, et al. Incidence, clinical characteristics and outcome of congestive heart failure as the initial presentation in patients with primary hyperthyroidism. Heart 2007;93:483–7.

Novel Biological Therapies Targeting Heart Failure: Myocardial Rejuvenation

 CrossMark

Amanda J. Favreau-Lessard, PhD, Sergey Ryzhov, MD, PhD,
Douglas B. Sawyer, MD, PhD*

KEYWORDS

- Heart failure • Rejuvenation • Cell therapy • Gene therapy

KEY POINTS

- Therapies targeting myocardial rejuvenation represent a promising area of investigation for advanced heart failure.
- Bone marrow–derived and cardiac-derived mesenchymal stem cells have exhibited some promising results, although further investigation is needed.
- Scarring and fibrosis, which occur in some forms of heart failure, require a search for ways to reprogram fibroblasts, or find strategies to rebuild cardiac tissue.
- Developmentally critical cell-signaling factors, such as NRG1β, SDF-1, or FSTL1, offer possible strategies to manipulate cardiac repair and rejuvenation.
- Gene delivery strategies are improving, allowing for induction of cardiac-specific expression of proteins involved in improving mechanical function, such as SERCA or Pim1.

INTRODUCTION

The great man is he who does not lose his child-like heart
—Mencius, Confucian Philosopher, ca 300 BC

Cardiovascular disease (CVD) is the leading cause of death across the globe, accounting for 17.3 million deaths per year.[1] In the United States, more than 1 in 3 adults suffers from some form of cardiovascular disease (85.6 million people), with 15.5 million experiencing coronary heart disease (CHD).[1] Among the types of CHD, 5.7 million people have heart failure (HF).[1] These statistics highlight the epidemic that is continually growing among the global population. Current therapies for HF with reduced ejection fraction focus on preserving left ventricular function as well as restoring cardiac function through the use of mechanical circulatory support devices or, in select patients, heart transplantation. The enormous growth in our understanding of heart biology as well as pathobiology leading to HF over the past several decades promises novel therapeutic approaches that will harness this biology to restore heart function.

Myocardial regeneration to some is the "holy grail" of HF translational research. Organ regeneration is an ancient concept. One of the most well-known stories of organ regeneration dates back to Greek mythology, where the Titan Prometheus, as punishment for deceiving Zeus, was forever chained to a rock where an eagle came each day to dine on his liver. Each evening his liver regenerated, whereupon the next day the eagle returned to continue its punishment. It is now well known that the adult liver indeed has remarkable regenerative potential, as does the bone marrow. The regenerative potential of the heart has also been recently established, at least

Center for Molecular Medicine, Maine Medical Center Research Institute, Maine Medical Center, 81 Research Drive, Scarborough, ME 04074, USA
* Corresponding author.
E-mail address: DSawyer@mmc.org

Heart Failure Clin 12 (2016) 461–471
http://dx.doi.org/10.1016/j.hfc.2016.03.008
1551-7136/16/$ – see front matter © 2016 Elsevier Inc. All rights reserved.

in lower vertebrates and young mammals.[2,3] When the chest of a young zebrafish or mouse is carefully opened, and the apical segment of the ventricular myocardium is clipped away, some organisms will survive through a process of growing new myocardium in its place. This process involved mesenchymal stem cells proliferating and differentiating in an organized way to replace the missing heart muscle in young animals. The adult heart throughout life responds to injury and stress with activated expression of genes involved in cardiac development, the so-called fetal gene program. In addition, both mesenchymal and bone marrow–derived progenitor cells are activated by cardiac injury. And yet, these processes are inadequate to restore heart function. Therapeutic approaches that manipulate these signals and processes are the cornerstone of biologic therapies for HF.

Based on the ancient wisdom of the Confucian scholar, the "Mencius Paradigm" is a term we have coined to characterize the hypothesis that biologic signals and processes critical for cardiac development might be manipulated to improve adult heart function. In this context, we propose that the term myocardial "rejuvenation," rather than "regeneration," is a more realistic outcome of these clinically motivated translational research efforts. In this brief review, we describe the state of a number of approaches at various stages of development using biologics, many of which fit the Mencius Paradigm.

CELL-BASED THERAPIES FOR HEART FAILURE WITH REDUCED EJECTION FRACTION

Developmental biology research has created detailed knowledge over how pluripotent cell lineages differentiate in an organized and highly programmed way to become the functional heart. The recognition that progenitor or stem cells which can differentiate into cardiac cells exist both in the bone marrow as well as the myocardium has led to a number of completed and ongoing experimental efforts asking if these can be used to restore ventricular function. Although in general the results are encouraging, it appears we are still some distance away from applying these strategies in the clinic. We outline a few of the stem cell-based approaches describing how specific cell types are being examined as potential therapy for HF.

Bone Marrow–Derived Mesenchymal Stem Cells

Mesenchymal stem cells (MSCs) are thought to be one of the most promising cell-based therapies for cardiovascular disease. Bone marrow–derived (BM-) MSCs can differentiate into many mature cardiac cell types, including cardiomyocytes, cardiac fibroblasts, and smooth muscle cells.[4–6] This makes BM-MSCs attractive for cell-based therapies to treat cardiac injury and HF. Under the proper conditions, these cells will differentiate into multiple lineages, hence it is hypothesized that by providing these cells to the heart by direct injection they will develop into functional cells that promote cardiac repair and restoration of heart function (for more in-depth review see Refs.[7,8]). MSCs have been well reported to migrate to an injured site to promote repair by immune modulation through a secretome.[9,10] The MSC secretome is also thought to play an important role in MSC repair. The secretome includes cytokines, such as interleukins, growth hormones, and exosomes, containing factors including microRNAs.[9,10] Thus, these cells may enable rejuvenation at sites of cardiac injury through differentiation into new cardiac cells, as well as provision of the necessary factors to aide repair. BM-MSCs are being examined in clinical trials (**Table 1**) with some evidence of success.[11–13]

Cardiac-Derived Mesenchymal Stem Cells

In recent years, subsets of cells within the heart, rather than the bone marrow, have been characterized as "cardiac stem cells" or "cardiac progenitor cells" due to their unique multipotent properties. Endogenous cardiac progenitor cells, also known as cardiac-derived MSCs, have been characterized by their ability to differentiate to cardiac cell types, including endothelial cells, fibroblasts, and myofibroblasts.[18–23] Directing differentiation of progenitors toward cardiac myocytes and limiting their conversion into non-myocyte cells, specifically fibroblasts/myofibroblasts, is an attractive approach to regenerate cardiac tissue after injury.[24] Two markers, adult stem cell antigen-1 (Sca-1) and c-Kit, are widely used to identify progenitors within CD45-negative nonhematopoietic cells in adult murine heart. The c-kit$^+$CD45$^-$ cells, which are also found in the human heart, are undergoing clinical trials to repair cardiac injury.[25,26] Sca-1 positive murine cardiac progenitors have been characterized as small interstitial cells located adjacent to the basal lamina and in proximity with CD31-positive endothelial cells (EC),[27] indicating a close relationship between EC and progenitor cells. Additional characteristics of this population are strong cell surface expression of CD105 and low or negative expression of CD31/PECAM1 and absence of CD34 and CD45 hematopoietic cell markers. No expression of c-Kit was found on these cells.[22] Human cardiac

Table 1
Clinical trials for mesenchymal stem cell therapy for heart failure

Study	ClinicalTrials.gov Identifier	Phase	Status	Outcomes
Autologous Mesenchymal Stromal Cell Therapy in Heart Failure	NCT00644410	Phase I/II	Completed	Therapy by intramyocardial injection of MSCs was safe and improved ejection fraction by >6% compared to placebo.[14]
Efficacy and Safety of Allogeneic Mesenchymal Precursor Cells for the Treatment of Chronic Heart Failure	NCT02032004	Phase III	Recruiting	N/A, estimated study completion is August 2018.
Transendocardial Delivery of Allogeneic Mesenchymal Precursor Cells (MPCs) in Heart Failure	NCT00721045	Phase II	Completed	No publication or results currently reported.
Safety and Efficacy of Intracoronary Adult Human Mesenchymal Stem Cells After Acute Myocardial Infarction (SEED-MSC)	NCT01392105	Phase II/III	Completed	One mo after patients with MI received MSC treatment; at 6 mo post-MI there was a slight improvement in LVEF; treatment was safe and there were no significant complications.[15]
Intravenous Dose of (aMBMC) to Subjects With Non-ischemic Heart Failure	NCT02467387	Phase II	Recruiting	N/A, estimated study completion is April 2017.
Transendocardial Autologous Cells (hMSC or hBMC) in Ischemic Heart Failure Trial (TAC-HFT)	NCT00768066	Phase I/II	Completed	Transendocardial injection of MSCs appeared safe, but due to sample size, distinct conclusions were difficult to elucidate; results provided evidence for larger-cohort investigations.[16]
Transendocardial Autologous Cells (hMSC or hMSC and hCSC) in Ischemic Heart Failure Trial (TAC-HFT II)	NCT02503280	Phase I/II	Not open yet to recruiting	N/A
Safety Study of Adult Mesenchymal Stem Cells (MSC) to Treat Acute Myocardial Infarction	NCT00114452	Phase I	Completed	No publication or results currently reported but an associated preclinical study in a swine MI model showed attenuation of contractile dysfunction in pigs treated with MSCs.[17]
Mesenchymal Stem Cells and Myocardial Ischemia (MESAMI)	NCT01076920	Phase I/II	Completed	No publication or results currently reported.

Abbreviations: LVEF, left ventricular ejection fraction; MI, myocardial infarction; N/A; Not available; SC, mesenchymal stem cell.

CD105$^+$ CD31$^-$ c-Kit$^-$ cells have been characterized by ability to differentiate toward cardiac myocytes.[22]

Cardiac progenitors are thought to be in a quiescent state until they are activated for proliferation and differentiation following injury to the heart. The major issue with these cells being used as therapy for cardiac repair is their limited number within the heart. An alternative strategy would be to find a way to specifically activate these cells to proliferate and differentiate to functional cardiomyocytes in the damaged area. Cardiac progenitors have been shown to promote myocardial regeneration after myocardial injury.[21] Factors that have been shown to alter these cells' ability to proliferate and differentiate include paracrine factors such as cytokines and growth hormones, exosomes/microvesicles, and microRNA. For example, miR-133a has been reported to promote protection of cardiac progenitors after myocardial ischemia by inhibiting proapoptotic factors and promoting cell survival.[28] Inhibition of profibrotic factors promotes cardioprotection of cardiac progenitors by paracrine and autocrine action.[29] Through paracrine signaling of insulin-like growth factor-1 (IGF-1), one study reports cardioprotection of cardiac progenitors, with improved cardiomyocyte survival and contractility.[30] A Phase I/II trial (ClinicalTrials.gov Identifier: NCT01438086) is currently recruiting patients to the RESUS-AMI study titled "Evaluation of the Safety and Efficacy of Using Insulin-like Growth Factor-1 in Patients With a Heart Attack."

Multiple Stem Cell Therapies

A new area of interest in cell based therapies is treatment with a mixture of multiple cell types. This is thought of as "second-generation" cell-based therapy, and although similar to BM-MSC therapies, differs as it is a calculated mixture of stem cells instead of a patient's isolated BM-MSCs. One cell combination that appears promising for cardiac repair is a mixture of c-kit$^+$ cardiac progenitor cells with BM-MSCs.[31] These cells are very similar in that they differentiate to the same types of mature cardiac stem cells but are beneficial for different properties. These mixed cell therapies are referred to as CardioChimeras where these cells are generated ex vivo via viral cell fusion.[32] MSCs, as previously described, have paracrine effects that limit inflammation, and promote survival and growth of adjacent cells.[9] The cardiac progenitors appear to promote regeneration.[32,33] To date, CardioChimeras have been tested only in preclinical models, where after myocardial infarction their use was associated

with reduced infarct size and improved cardiac function.[32] There is one clinical trial currently recruiting patients to test the effects of MSC and cardiac stem cell therapies alone or in combination in patients with HF (CONCERT-HF, clinicaltrials. gov identifier: NCT02501811).

REPROGRAMMING SCARRING

Scar formation and fibrosis represent a major problem for cardiac regeneration and rejuvenation efforts after cardiac injury. Recent work has explored strategies to reverse scarring via reprogramming. Using genetic manipulation strategies, investigators have identified key factors that can be targeted to undifferentiated myofibroblasts so as to reprogram cells to form functional heart muscle and limit fibrosis. One strategy under investigation is reprogramming cardiac fibroblasts into functional cardiomyocyte-like cells. By locally delivering developmentally critical transcription factors (Gata4, Mef2c, and Tbx5) to the infarcted area, cardiac fibroblasts were reprogrammed into binucleated cardiomyocyte-like cells with mechanical and electrical coupling to existing cardiac myocytes.[34] This approach also decreased the size of the infarct zone and modestly attenuated cardiac dysfunction in the months following injury.[34] Addition of thymosin b4 to the transcription factor mix further improved cardiac function and scarring.[34] Although this approach remains at the preclinical-phase of development, the demonstration that fibroblasts can be reprogrammed represents a promising therapeutic avenue.

STIMULATING MYOCYTE CELL CYCLE REENTRY

Cardiac myocytes build the myocardium during development and complete growth of the heart during adolescence as the cardiomyocytes reach mature size and structure. Cardiac myocytes within the heart have very little turnover throughout life. Because cardiac myocytes are fundamental to heart function, a method to promote these cells to reenter the cell cycle through dedifferentiation followed by proliferation and formation of new functional cardiac myocytes following cardiac damage is an area of therapeutic interest (for more information on this topic, see Ref.[35]). In one example, studies with in vivo and in vitro treatment of oncostatin M, an inflammatory cytokine of the interleukin IL-6 family, dedifferentiates cardiac myocytes and promotes cardiac protection of the myocardium.[36,37] Cardiac myocytes reenter the cell cycle and proliferate after periostin treatment, which activates integrins and the PI3K pathway.[38] When provided as treatment in an in vivo model of myocardial infarction, long-term delivery of periostin through an epicardial patch improved cardiac function, reduced fibrosis, and reduced hypertrophy.[38] Interestingly, stimulation with neuregulin-1 (NRG-1, described in more detail later in this article) promotes cardiac myocyte dedifferentiation and proliferation both in vitro and in vivo.[39] Additionally, in vivo treatment of NRG-1 in mice following cardiac injury resulted in myocardial regeneration and repair.[39] Targeting cardiac myocyte proliferation through factors such as these or in conjunction with factors discussed in the two sections below on promoting myocardial rejuvenation could protect the myocardium when injured or promote myocardial repair following injury.

MANIPULATING CELL SIGNALING TO PROMOTE MYOCARDIAL REJUVENATION

A number of recombinant proteins have been explored as potential treatments for HF. Growth factors with roles in heart development or cardiomyocyte differentiation top the list and are discussed later in this article (**Table 2**). Other factors not listed in the table but worthy of mentioning include IGF-1, fibroblast growth factors, and vascular endothelial growth factor (VEGF). IGF-1 promotes cardiac stem cell repair and activates pro-survival pathways.[40] Fibroblast growth factors (FGFs), such as FGF9, improve contractile function following myocardial infarction and promote myocardial vascularization.[41]

Neuregulin 1 Beta

Neuregulin (NRG) is a developmentally critical growth factor that works through inducing ErbB-receptor tyrosine kinase activation and subsequent downstream signaling pathways. The NRG-1β isoform of NRG has effects on cardiomyocyte survival as well as structure and function in vitro, in addition to endothelial cell and fibroblast responses.[42,43] In addition, NRG-1β activates differentiation of progenitor cell populations toward cardiac cell lineages, at least in vitro.[44,45] Some or all of these effects may explain how recombinant NRG-1β given to both animals and humans with systolic dysfunction is associated with improvements in heart function. There are two distinct recombinant NRG-1β proteins in clinical development. The epidermal growth factor (EGF)-domain–only fragment of NRG-1β has progressed to late-stage clinical trials[46,47] (for more detail, see Ref.[48]). When given as a parenteral infusion over many days, a sustained improvement in cardiac function has been reported.[47] The larger recombinant glial growth factor 2 (GGF2), which is a naturally expressed type II NRG-1β isoform, is effective in improving cardiac function in small and large animals.[49,50] Early results in humans have been presented[51,52] (for more detail, see Ref.[53]).

Stromal Cell–Derived Factor 1

Stromal cell–derived factor 1 (SDF-1) is a chemokine involved in cell recruitment. Within the heart, CXCR4 is the primary receptor that SDF-1 acts through and promotes cell homing, remodeling, and cardiomyocyte survival.[54,55] After myocardial ischemia, SDF-1 treatment increases migration and recruits progenitor cells to sites of cardiac damage.[56–58] A multifunctional fusion protein of SDF-1 and glycoprotein VI given after myocardial infarction induced recruitment of bone marrow cells to the damaged myocardium and reduced infarct size.[59] Thus, SDF-1 treatment may complement stem cell–based therapies through enhancing cell homing and promoting remodeling. Clinical trials using gene therapy for overexpression of SDF-1 are continuing to be investigated for therapeutic potential.[54]

Follistatin-related Protein 1

Follistatin-related protein 1 (FSTL1) is a glycoprotein expressed within the epicardium that inhibits TGFβ signaling. In myocardial ischemia, BMP4 and phosphorylated SMADs 1/5/8 are elevated in the heart but with FSTL1 treatment phosphorylated SMAD1/5/8 levels are attenuated.[60] Recombinant human FSTL1 delivered via epicardial patch after myocardial infarction activated cardiomyocyte cell cycle reentry and subsequent division of preexisting cardiomyocytes, in association with improved cardiac function and survival.[61,62] Interestingly, transgenic overexpression of FSTL1 in this study did not lead to improved cardiac function or survival.[61,62] This phenomenon is thought to be dependent on the location or origin of FSTL1, which may affect the glycosylation of the protein and provide a different response. Preclinical investigations are ongoing to determine the proper delivery strategy of FSTL1 for clinical trial studies.

Biologic Vasodilators

Natriuretic peptides are also considered part of the "fetal gene program," with strong activation of expression on cardiac injury or stress. Physiologically, these peptides induce vasodilation and sodium excretion, while antagonizing the effects of angiotensin II and aldosterone through activation of guanylate cyclase (GC) receptors A and B. Recombinant natriuretic peptides that have been developed to treat HF, such as nesiritide

Table 2
Gene targets for heart failure therapy

Biological Factor	Mechanism of Action	In Vivo Support
NRG-1β (EGF-domain only and GGF2 isoforms)	Multiple mechanisms including cardiac myocyte structure, function, and survival; suppression of fibrosis and inflammation.	• Swine with myocardial infarction treated with GGF2 have reduced fibrosis in association with improved left ventricular remodeling and contractile function.[49] • Rats with myocardial infarction treated with GGF2 exhibit improved left ventricular function.[50] • Clinical trials with EGF-domain recombinant human NRG-1 have shown improvement in left ventricular ejection fraction in patients with chronic heart failure.[47] • Early clinical trials of the GGF2 isoform of NRG-1 indicate the safety of this therapy and demonstrate similar success as to the EGF-domain recombinant human NRG-1 therapy.[51,52]
SERCA	Improves calcium dynamics.	• Transgenic SERCA1a hearts following myocardial ischemia have improved contractility and reduced infarct size compared with nontransgenic hearts.[73] • SERCA2a gene therapy in a chronic heart failure rat model exhibited stabilized sarcoplasmic reticulum calcium load and reduced spontaneous and catecholamine-induced ventricular arrhythmias.[74] • Despite promising results from proof-of-concept studies, intracoronary infusion of AAV1/SERCA2a did not improve the clinical course of patients with heart failure and reduced ejection fraction.[75,76]
Pim1	Inhibition of cardiomyocyte cell death and enhanced calcium dynamics.	• Transgenic Pim1 mice exhibited cardiac protection from myocardial infarction through inhibition of cardiomyocyte apoptosis as well as improved calcium dynamics through elevated SERCA2a expression.[77] • Injection of human cardiac progenitor cells overexpressing Pim1 kinase into mice after myocardial infarction improved cardiac function and structure with reduced infarct.[78]
SDF-1	Promotes migration of progenitor cells to sites of injury.	• SDF-1 promotes recruitment of progenitor cells to sites of cardiac damage following myocardial ischemia.[56,57] • A bifunctional protein of SDF-1 and glycoprotein VI tested in a mouse model of myocardial infarction increased recruitment of bone marrow cells to the infarct area, which reduced infarct size and preserved cardiac function.[59]

(continued on next page)

Table 2
(continued)

Biological Factor	Mechanism of Action	In Vivo Support
miR-15	Suppresses myocyte proliferation and viability.	• Inhibition of miR-15 increases systolic function and myocyte proliferation following myocardial infarction in mice.[82] • miR-15 inhibition increases viability of cardiomyocytes, decreases fibrosis, improves ejection fraction and reduces infarct size following ischemia-reperfusion injury.[81]
FSTL1	Stimulates myocyte proliferation.	• Human FSTL1 epicardial patch improves cardiac function and survival in swine and mouse myocardial injury models.[61,62]

Abbreviations: AAV1, adeno-associated virus 1; EGF, epidermal growth factor; FSTL1, follistatin-related protein 1; GGF2, glial growth factor 2; NRG-1, neuregulin-1; Pim1, proto-oncogene serine/threonine-protein kinase; SDF-I, stromal cell–derived factor 1; SERCA, sarcoplasmic reticulum Ca^{2+} ATPase.

(recombinant B-type natriuretic peptide [BNP]), have lost traction in clinical practice.[63] New natriuretic peptides and other vasodilators with additional biological properties are being developed to improve HF outcomes. Atrial natriuretic peptide (aka A-type NP, ANP) remains under investigation.[64] Cendiritide (CD-NP) is a recombinant engineered natriuretic peptide that combines elements of naturally occurring C-type and D-type NP, which optimizes its agonist action on both GC-A and CG-B,[65] and may have unique antifibrotic activity. Combined with bioengineered scaffolds and other drug-delivery methods, this novel peptide holds particular promise for vascular as well as myocardial disease.[66,67]

One promising non-natriuretic peptide vasodilator is the placenta-derived factor relaxin, which mediates cardiovascular adaptation to pregnancy. In addition to its potent action as a vasodilator, relaxin regulates extracellular matrix and remodeling, increases angiogenesis, and improves function after ischemic injury.[68,69] Serelaxin, a recombinant human relaxin-2, has been studied in humans with acute HF, where it is tolerated,[70] and in a larger international trial has been associated with symptomatic relief.[71] Serelaxin remains under investigation primarily for the treatment of acute HF. For more information on this topic, we suggest Refs.[68,72].

MANIPULATING GENE EXPRESSION TO PROMOTE MYOCARDIAL REJUVENATION
Sarcoplasmic Reticulum Ca^{2+} ATPase

The expression of sarcoplasmic reticulum Ca^{2+} ATPase (SERCA), essential to electrical-mechanical coupling in cardiac myocytes, is sensitive to cardiac injury. Reduction of SERCA2a activity is correlated with a variety of cardiac disease states, including HF. In a variety of animal models of HF, increasing expression of SERCA restores Ca^{2+} handling, improves contractility, and reduces cardiac injury.[73,74] This has led to an ongoing effort using an adeno-associated viral vector to restore myocardial expression of SERCA2a. Although a small phase 2 trial demonstrated improvement in clinical parameters, as well as cardiac function,[75] these were not reproduced in a larger phase 2 trial.[76] Further clinical trials will be necessary to determine whether this approach can be of benefit to patients with HF. However, important advances made during this program's development include those made in viral vectors for use in gene therapy.

Proto-Oncogene Serine/Threonine-Protein Kinase

Proto-oncogene serine/threonine-protein kinase (Pim1) is an enzyme involved in cell cycle, transcriptional activation, and apoptosis. Within the heart, Pim1 overexpression has been shown to protect the heart from myocardial infarction through increasing SERCA2a expression, thereby improving calcium dynamics and promoting cardiomyocyte survival.[77] Using a mouse model of myocardial infarction, injection of human cardiac progenitors into the heart that overexpressed Pim1 resulted in improved cardiac function with reduced myocardial damage and elevated homing of treatment progenitor cells.[78] Studies of Pim1 have also shown beneficial effects on the myocardium through promoting contractility of myocytes and enhancing the proliferative effects of cardiac progenitors,[79] thus providing evidence that Pim1 could be used as HF therapy.

miR-15

MicroRNAs are small noncoding nucleotides that regulate transcript and protein of their target genes through mRNA inhibition or degradation. The specific microRNA miR-15 increases in expression in the heart after injury and inhibits the TGFβ signaling pathway resulting in increased fibrosis.[80] Functionally, inhibition of miR-15 in vivo in a myocardial infarction model increases the viability of cardiomyocytes and increases differentiation.[81,82] Thus, miR-15 has been proposed as a target following cardiac injury to promote cardiomyocyte vitality and growth.[83] Although this strategy remains in preclinical development, microRNAs in general represent an exciting area of investigation as potential targets for HF therapies.

SUMMARY

Biological therapeutics are an exciting area of development with potential to change the dynamics of HF therapy. Although there has been much written about myocardial regeneration, we believe that "rejuvenation" is perhaps a better term to describe the desired state of reverse remodeling and ventricular recovery for patients with HF. Despite decades of research, this field is still in its "infancy", pun intended. A promising direction is the continued investigation of signals and events in cardiac development and the progressive study of interesting leads that might promote myocardial rejuvenation after injury in the adult heart. Thus, further investigation is needed by both developmental biologists as well as translational scientists to fully explore the Mencius Paradigm and bring biological therapies for advanced HF to fruition.

REFERENCES

1. Mozaffarian D, Benjamin EJ, Go AS, et al. Heart disease and stroke statistics–2015 update: a report from the American Heart Association. Circulation 2015;131:e29–322.
2. Porrello ER, Mahmoud AI, Simpson E, et al. Transient regenerative potential of the neonatal mouse heart. Science 2011;331:1078–80.
3. Poss KD, Wilson LG, Keating MT. Heart regeneration in zebrafish. Science 2002;298:2188–90.
4. Xu W, Zhang X, Qian H, et al. Mesenchymal stem cells from adult human bone marrow differentiate into a cardiomyocyte phenotype in vitro. Exp Biol Med (Maywood) 2004;229:623–31.
5. Tamama K, Sen CK, Wells A. Differentiation of bone marrow mesenchymal stem cells into the smooth muscle lineage by blocking ERK/MAPK signaling pathway. Stem Cells Dev 2008;17:897–908.
6. Souders CA, Bowers SL, Baudino TA. Cardiac fibroblast: the renaissance cell. Circ Res 2009;105:1164–76.
7. Williams AR, Hare JM. Mesenchymal stem cells: biology, pathophysiology, translational findings, and therapeutic implications for cardiac disease. Circ Res 2011;109:923–40.
8. Pittenger MF, Martin BJ. Mesenchymal stem cells and their potential as cardiac therapeutics. Circ Res 2004;95:9–20.
9. Wang Y, Chen X, Cao W, et al. Plasticity of mesenchymal stem cells in immunomodulation: pathological and therapeutic implications. Nat Immunol 2014;15:1009–16.
10. Ranganath SH, Levy O, Inamdar MS, et al. Harnessing the mesenchymal stem cell secretome for the treatment of cardiovascular disease. Cell Stem Cell 2012;10:244–58.
11. Mathiasen AB, Qayyum AA, Jørgensen E, et al. Bone marrow-derived mesenchymal stromal cell treatment in patients with severe ischaemic heart failure: a randomized placebo-controlled trial (MSC-HF trial). Eur Heart J 2015;36:1744–53.
12. Lee JW, Lee SH, Youn YJ, et al. A randomized, open-label, multicenter trial for the safety and efficacy of adult mesenchymal stem cells after acute myocardial infarction. J Korean Med Sci 2014;29:23–31.
13. Heldman AW, DiFede DL, Fishman JE, et al. Transendocardial mesenchymal stem cells and mononuclear bone marrow cells for ischemic cardiomyopathy: the TAC-HFT randomized trial. JAMA 2014;311:62–73.
14. Shake JG, Gruber PJ, Baumgartner WA, et al. Mesenchymal stem cell implantation in a swine myocardial infarct model: engraftment and functional effects. Ann Thorac Surg 2002;73:1919–25 [discussion: 1926].
15. Narita T, Suzuki K. Bone marrow-derived mesenchymal stem cells for the treatment of heart failure. Heart Fail Rev 2015;20:53–68.
16. Sanina C, Hare JM. Mesenchymal stem cells as a biological drug for heart disease: where are we with cardiac cell-based therapy? Circ Res 2015;117:229–33.
17. Karantalis V, Hare JM. Use of mesenchymal stem cells for therapy of cardiac disease. Circ Res 2015;116:1413–30.
18. Smith RR, Barile L, Cho HC, et al. Regenerative potential of cardiosphere-derived cells expanded from percutaneous endomyocardial biopsy specimens. Circulation 2007;115:896–908.

19. Beltrami AP, Barlucchi L, Torella D, et al. Adult cardiac stem cells are multipotent and support myocardial regeneration. Cell 2003;114:763–76.

20. Rota M, Padin-Iruegas ME, Misao Y, et al. Local activation or implantation of cardiac progenitor cells rescues scarred infarcted myocardium improving cardiac function. Circ Res 2008;103:107–16.

21. Ellison GM, Vicinanza C, Smith AJ, et al. Adult c-kit(pos) cardiac stem cells are necessary and sufficient for functional cardiac regeneration and repair. Cell 2013;154:827–42.

22. Ryzhov S, Goldstein AE, Novitskiy SV, et al. Role of A2B adenosine receptors in regulation of paracrine functions of stem cell antigen 1-positive cardiac stromal cells. J Pharmacol Exp Ther 2012; 341:764–74.

23. Ryzhov S, Sung BH, Zhang Q, et al. Role of adenosine a receptor signaling in contribution of cardiac mesenchymal stem-like cells to myocardial scar formation. Purinergic Signal 2014;10(3):477–86.

24. van Berlo JH, Molkentin JD. An emerging consensus on cardiac regeneration. Nat Med 2014;20:1386–93.

25. Bolli R, Chugh AR, D'Amario D, et al. Cardiac stem cells in patients with ischaemic cardiomyopathy (SCIPIO): initial results of a randomised phase 1 trial. Lancet 2011;378:1847–57.

26. Makkar RR, Smith RR, Cheng K, et al. Intracoronary cardiosphere-derived cells for heart regeneration after myocardial infarction (CADUCEUS): a prospective, randomised phase 1 trial. Lancet 2012;379: 895–904.

27. Oh H, Bradfute SB, Gallardo TD, et al. Cardiac progenitor cells from adult myocardium: homing, differentiation, and fusion after infarction. Proc Natl Acad Sci U S A 2003;100:12313–8.

28. Izarra A, Moscoso I, Levent E, et al. Mir-133a enhances the protective capacity of cardiac progenitors cells after myocardial infarction. Stem Cell Reports 2014;3:1029–42.

29. Ho YS, Tsai WH, Lin FC, et al. Cardioprotective actions of TGFbetaRI inhibition through stimulating autocrine/paracrine of survivin and inhibiting Wnt in cardiac progenitors. Stem Cells 2015;34(2): 445–55.

30. Kawaguchi N, Smith AJ, Waring CD, et al. C-kitpos GATA-4 high rat cardiac stem cells foster adult cardiomyocyte survival through IGF-1 paracrine signalling. PLoS One 2010;5:e14297.

31. Williams AR, Hatzistergos KE, Addicott B, et al. Enhanced effect of combining human cardiac stem cells and bone marrow mesenchymal stem cells to reduce infarct size and to restore cardiac function after myocardial infarction. Circulation 2013;127: 213–23.

32. Quijada P, Salunga HT, Hariharan N, et al. Cardiac stem cell hybrids enhance myocardial repair. Circ Res 2015;117:695–706.

33. Leri A, Kajstura J, Anversa P. Cardiac stem cells and mechanisms of myocardial regeneration. Physiol Rev 2005;85:1373–416.

34. Qian L, Huang Y, Spencer CI, et al. In vivo reprogramming of murine cardiac fibroblasts into induced cardiomyocytes. Nature 2012;485:593–8.

35. Senyo SE, Lee RT, Kuhn B. Cardiac regeneration based on mechanisms of cardiomyocyte proliferation and differentiation. Stem Cell Res 2014;13: 532–41.

36. Kubin T, Pöling J, Kostin S, et al. Oncostatin M is a major mediator of cardiomyocyte dedifferentiation and remodeling. Cell Stem Cell 2011;9:420–32.

37. Poling J, Gajawada P, Richter M, et al. Therapeutic targeting of the oncostatin M receptor-beta prevents inflammatory heart failure. Basic Res Cardiol 2014; 109:396.

38. Kuhn B, del Monte F, Hajjar RJ, et al. Periostin induces proliferation of differentiated cardiomyocytes and promotes cardiac repair. Nat Med 2007;13: 962–9.

39. Bersell K, Arab S, Haring B, et al. Neuregulin1/ ErbB4 signaling induces cardiomyocyte proliferation and repair of heart injury. Cell 2009;138:257–70.

40. Galindo CL, Kasasbeh E, Murphy A, et al. Anti-remodeling and anti-fibrotic effects of the neuregulin-1beta glial growth factor 2 in a large animal model of heart failure. J Am Heart Assoc 2014; 3:e000773.

41. Jabbour A, Zhang J, Cheng L, et al. Parenteral administration of recombinant human neuregulin-1 to patients with stable chronic heart failure produces favourable acute and chronic haemodynamic responses. Eur J Heart Fail 2011;13:83–92.

42. Brittain E, Muldowney J, Geisberg C, et al. Evaluation of cardiac function in symptomatic heart failure patients in a single infusion, phase 1, dose escalation study of glial growth factor 2. J Am Coll Cardiol 2013;61.

43. Lenihan DJ, Anderson S, Geisberg C, et al. Safety and tolerability of glial growth factor 2 in patients with chronic heart failure: a phase I single dose escalation study. J Am Coll Cardiol 2013;61.

44. Lyon AR, Bannister ML, Collins T, et al. SERCA2a gene transfer decreases sarcoplasmic reticulum calcium leak and reduces ventricular arrhythmias in a model of chronic heart failure. Circ Arrhythm Electrophysiol 2011;4:362–72.

45. Jessup M, Greenberg B, Mancini D, et al. Calcium upregulation by percutaneous administration of gene therapy in cardiac disease (CUPID): a phase 2 trial of intracoronary gene therapy of sarcoplasmic reticulum Ca2+-ATPase in patients with advanced heart failure. Circulation 2011;124:304–13.

46. Greenberg B, Butler J, Felker GM, et al. Calcium upregulation by percutaneous administration of gene therapy in patients with cardiac disease

(CUPID 2): a randomised, multinational, double-blind, placebo-controlled, phase 2b trial. Lancet 2016. http://dx.doi.org/10.1016/S0140-6736(16)00082-9.

47. Muraski JA, Rota M, Misao Y, et al. Pim-1 regulates cardiomyocyte survival downstream of Akt. Nat Med 2007;13:1467–75.

48. Mohsin S, Khan M, Toko H, et al. Human cardiac progenitor cells engineered with Pim-I kinase enhance myocardial repair. J Am Coll Cardiol 2012;60:1278–87.

49. Askari AT, Unzek S, Popovic ZB, et al. Effect of stromal-cell-derived factor 1 on stem-cell homing and tissue regeneration in ischaemic cardio-myopathy. Lancet 2003;362:697–703.

50. Cheng M, Huang K, Zhou J, et al. A critical role of Src family kinase in SDF-1/CXCR4-mediated bone-marrow progenitor cell recruit-ment to the ischemic heart. J Mol Cell Cardiol 2015;81:49–53.

51. Ziegler M, Elvers M, Baumer Y, et al. The bispecific SDF1-GPVI fusion protein preserves myocardial function after transient ischemia in mice. Circulation 2012;125:685–96.

52. Porrello ER, Mahmoud AI, Simpson E, et al. Regula-tion of neonatal and adult mammalian heart regener-ation by the miR-15 family. Proc Natl Acad Sci U S A 2013;110:187–92.

53. Hullinger TG, Montgomery RL, Seto AG, et al. Inhibi-tion of miR-15 protects against cardiac ischemic injury. Circ Res 2012;110:71–81.

54. Wei K, Serpooshan V, Hurtado C, et al. Epicardial FSTL1 reconstitution regenerates the adult mamma-lian heart. Nature 2015;525:479–85.

55. van Rooij E. Cardiac repair after myocardial infarc-tion. N Engl J Med 2016;374:85–7.

56. Jackson R, Tilokee EL, Latham N, et al. Paracrine engineering of human cardiac stem cells with insulin-like growth factor 1 enhances myocardial repair. J Am Heart Assoc 2015;4:e002104.

57. Korf-Klingebiel M, Kempf T, Schlüter KD, et al. Conditional transgenic expression of fibroblast growth factor 9 in the adult mouse heart reduces heart failure mortality after myocardial infarction. Circulation 2011;123:504–14.

58. Hill MF, Patel AV, Murphy A, et al. Intravenous glial growth factor 2 (GGF2) isoform of neuregulin-1beta improves left ventricular function, gene and protein expression in rats after myocardial infarction. PLoS One 2013;8:e55741.

59. Talukder MA, Kalyanasundaram A, Zhao X, et al. Expression of SERCA isoform with faster Ca2+ transport properties improves postischemic cardiac function and Ca2+ handling and decreases myocardial infarction. Am J Physiol Heart Circ Phys-iol 2007;293:H2418–28.

60. Kuramochi Y, Cote GM, Guo X, et al. Cardiac endothelial cells regulate reactive oxygen species-induced cardiomyocyte apoptosis through neuregulin-1beta/erbB4 signaling. J Biol Chem 2004;279:51141–7.

61. An T, Zhang Y, Huang Y, et al. Neuregulin-1 protects against doxorubicin-induced apoptosis in cardio-myocytes through an Akt-dependent pathway. Phys-iol Res 2013;62:379–85.

62. Iglesias-Garcia O, Baumgartner S, Macrí-Pellizzeri L, et al. Neuregulin-1beta induces mature ventricular cardiac differentiation from induced pluripotent stem cells contributing to cardiac tissue repair. Stem Cells Dev 2015;24:484–96.

63. Hao J, Galindo CL, Tran TL, et al. Neuregulin-1beta induces embryonic stem cell cardiomyogenesis via ErbB3/ErbB2 receptors. Biochem J 2014;458:335–41.

64. Gao R, Zhang J, Cheng L, et al. A Phase II, random-ized, double-blind, multicenter, based on standard therapy, placebo-controlled study of the efficacy and safety of recombinant human neuregulin-1 in patients with chronic heart failure. J Am Coll Cardiol 2010;55:1907–14.

65. Rupert CE, Coulombe KL. The roles of neuregulin-1 in cardiac development, homeostasis, and disease. Biomark Insights 2015;10:1–9.

66. Galindo CL, Ryzhov S, Sawyer DB. Neuregulin as a heart failure therapy and mediator of reverse remod-eling. Curr Heart Fail Rep 2014;11:40–9.

67. Penn MS, Pastore J, Miller T, et al. SDF-1 in myocar-dial repair. Gene Ther 2012;19:583–7.

68. Zaruba MM, Franz WM. Role of the SDF-1-CXCR4 axis in stem cell-based therapies for ischemic cardiomyopathy. Expert Opin Biol Ther 2010;10:321–35.

69. Wang K, Zhao X, Kuang C, et al. Overexpression of SDF-1alpha enhanced migration and engraft-ment of cardiac stem cells and reduced infarcted size via CXCR4/PI3K pathway. PLoS One 2012;7:e43922.

70. Ogura Y, Ouchi N, Ohashi K, et al. Therapeutic impact of follistatin-like 1 on myocardial ischemic injury in preclinical models. Circulation 2012;126:1728–38.

71. O'Connor CM, Starling RC, Hernandez AF, et al. Effect of nesiritide in patients with acute decom-pensated heart failure. N Engl J Med 2011;365:32–43.

72. Rubattu S, Calvieri C, Pagliaro B, et al. Atrial natri-uretic peptide and regulation of vascular function in hypertension and heart failure: implications for novel therapeutic strategies. J Hypertens 2013;31:1061–72.

73. Martin FL, Sangaralingham SJ, Huntley BK, et al. CD-NP: a novel engineered dual guanylyl cyclase activator with anti-fibrotic actions in the heart. PLoS One 2012;7:e52422.

74. Ng XW, Huang Y, Chen HH, et al. Cenderitide-eluting film for potential cardiac patch applications. PLoS One 2013;8:e68346.

75. Ng XW, Huang Y, Liu KL, et al. In vitro evaluation of cenderitide-eluting stent I—an antirestenosis and proendothelization approach. J Pharm Sci 2014; 103:3631–40.

76. Raleigh JM, Toldo S, Das A, et al. Relaxin' the heart: a novel therapeutic modality. J Cardiovasc Pharmacol Ther 2015. http://dx.doi.org/10.1177/1074248415617851.

77. Kumar VA, Wilson SS, Ayaz SI, et al. Targeted biological therapies reach the heart: the case of serelaxin for heart failure. Drugs Today (Barc) 2015;51:591–7.

78. Teerlink JR, Metra M, Felker GM, et al. Relaxin for the treatment of patients with acute heart failure (Pre-RELAX-AHF): a multicentre, randomised, placebo-controlled, parallel-group, dose-finding phase IIb study. Lancet 2009;373:1429–39.

79. Teerlink JR, Cotter G, Davison BA, et al. Serelaxin, recombinant human relaxin-2, for treatment of acute heart failure (RELAX-AHF): a randomised, placebo-controlled trial. Lancet 2013;381: 29–39.

80. Francis GS, Felker GM, Tang WH. A Test in context: critical evaluation of natriuretic peptide testing in heart failure. J Am Coll Cardiol 2016; 67:330–7.

81. Fischer KM, Cottage CT, Konstandin MH, et al. Pim-1 kinase inhibits pathological injury by promoting cardioprotective signaling. J Mol Cell Cardiol 2011; 51:554–8.

82. Tijsen AJ, van der Made I, van den Hoogenhof MM, et al. The microRNA-15 family inhibits the TGFbeta-pathway in the heart. Cardiovasc Res 2014;104:61–71.

83. Giacca M, Zacchigna S. Harnessing the microRNA pathway for cardiac regeneration. J Mol Cell Cardiol 2015;89:68–74.

Printed and bound by CPI Group (UK) Ltd, Croydon, CR0 4YY

03/10/2024

01040304-0007